DR. C.A. BENEDICT

Stronger Bones, Stronger You

A Complete Guide to Exercise for Osteoporosis and Discovering the Secrets to Building and Maintaining Healthy Bones at Any Age

First published by Dr. C.A. Benedict 2023

Copyright © 2023 by Dr. C.A. Benedict

All rights reserved. No part of this publication may be reproduced, stored or transmitted in any form or by any means, electronic, mechanical, photocopying, recording, scanning, or otherwise without written permission from the publisher. It is illegal to copy this book, post it to a website, or distribute it by any other means without permission.

Dr. C.A. Benedict asserts the moral right to be identified as the author of this work.

First edition

Advisor: N.G. Eucharia
Cover art by Thomas jasta poo

This book was professionally typeset on Reedsy.
Find out more at reedsy.com

Dedication.

To all those who have been diagnosed with osteoporosis and are determined to take control of their bone health through exercise, this book is dedicated to you. May it serve as a guide and a source of inspiration on your journey to stronger bones and a stronger you. Your strength and resilience are an inspiration to us all. I love you all!!!!

Contents

1 Chapter 1	1
Understanding Bone, and Osteoporosis:	1
Definition and causes of osteoporosis	3
Signs and symptoms of osteoporosis	7
Risk factors for developing osteoporosis	9
Complications of osteoporosis	12
2 Chapter 2	14
Why Exercise is Crucial for Osteoporosis?:	14
How exercise can help prevent and manage osteoporosis	14
Benefits of exercise for bone health	16
Types of exercises recommended for osteoporosis	18
How often and how much exercise is necessary for osteoporosis?	19
safety tips for your exercises and exercises you should avoid	20
Exercises You Should Avoid	22
3 Chapter 3	25
Building a Strong Foundation:	25
Assessing your current fitness level	27
Developing a safe and effective exercise plan	29
Starting slowly and gradually increasing intensity.	30
Finding support and guidance for your exercise routine	32
4 Chapter 4	35
Resistance Training:	35
Definition and benefits of resistance training:	35
Incorporating Resistance Training into an Osteoporosis Treatment Plan:	37

Examples of resistance exercises:	38
Squats:	38
Lunges:	39
Wall push-ups:	39
Seated rows:	39
Standing calf raises:	39
Daily routine plan and time table for resistance exercises:	40
Safety precautions for resistance training:	45
How to progress your resistance training:	47
5 Chapter 5	48
Weight-Bearing Exercises:	48
Definition and benefits of weight-bearing exercises	48
Benefits of weight-bearing exercises for osteoporosis	50
Examples of weight-bearing exercises	51
High impact weight bearing exercises; procedures and time table.	51
Jumping:	52
Dancing:	55
Running and jogging:	58
Hiking:	61
Stair climbing:	64
Safety precautions for weight-bearing exercises	65
How to progress your weight-bearing exercises	66
Low impact weight bearing exercises:	67
Walking:	68
Dancing:	68
Step aerobics:	68
Yoga:	68
Resistance training:	68
Daily routine plan and time table for walking exercises	69
Daily routine plan and time table for dancing exercises	70
Daily routine plan and time table for step acrobatics exercises	71
Daily routine plan and time table for yoga exercises	73

Daily routine plan and time table for resistance training exercises	74
6 Chapter 6	76
Definition and benefits of flexibility and balance exercises:	76
Types of flexibility exercises	76
Static stretching:	76
Daily routine plan for Static stretching exercises:	77
Dynamic stretching:	79
Passive stretching:	81
Daily routine plan for passive stretching exercises:	81
Active stretching:	83
Daily routine plan for active stretching exercises for an osteoporosis patient:	83
Benefits of flexibility exercises for osteoporosis patients:	85
Definition of balance exercises:	86
Types of balance exercises:	86
Standing balance exercises:	86
Dynamic balance exercises:	88
Proprioceptive training:	90
Benefits of balance exercises for osteoporosis patients:	92
Safety precautions for flexibility and balance training	94
How to progress your flexibility and balance exercises	95
Specific Exercises for Common	96
Hamstrings:	97
Hips:	97
Shoulders:	97
Core:	97
Ankles:	97
Knees:	97
Upper back:	98
7 Chapter 7	99
Exercises for a better posture and their procedures.	99
Shoulder blade squeeze	99
Wall angels:	100

Abdominal bracing:	101
Hip flexor stretch:	102
Walking:	103
Standing breaks:	104
8 Chapter 8	105
Osteoporosis-Related Injuries:	105
Fractures:	105
Compression fractures:	106
Hip fractures:	106
Wrist fractures:	106
Other injuries:	106
Exercises for Compression fractures:	107
Walking:	107
Tai Chi:	107
Water exercises:	107
Yoga:	108
Resistance training:	108
Exercises for hip fractures:	108
Exercises for vertebral fractures;	109
Exercises for wrist fractures:	110
Exercises for other common osteoporosis-related injuries:	111
9 Chapter 9	113
Overcoming Barriers to Exercise:	113
Common barriers to exercise and how to overcome them.	113
How to stay motivated to exercise:	115
Strategies for finding time to exercise:	116
Strategies for finding time to exercise:	117
How to adjust your exercise routine for physical limitations:	119
10 Chapter 10	121
Living Strong with Osteoporosis:	121
The importance of ongoing exercise for osteoporosis management:	121
The importance of ongoing exercise for osteoporosis management:	123
How to track your progress and set new goals	125

	Success stories of individuals with osteoporosis who have improved their bone health through exercise:	127
	Resources for continuing your osteoporosis exercise routine:	130
11	Chapter 11	133
	Lifestyle Changes to Support Bone Health:	133
	Nutrition for bone health:	133
	Calcium:	133
	Vitamin D:	134
	Magnesium:	134
	Vitamin K:	134
	Protein:	134
	Phosphorus:	134
	Other lifestyle changes that can support bone health	135
	The importance of calcium and vitamin D:	136
	Limiting risk factors for osteoporosis:	137
12	Conclusion	139

1

Chapter 1

Understanding Bone, and Osteoporosis:

Introduction:
Bones are complex, living tissues that provide support, protection, and mobility to the body. They are constantly undergoing a process of remodeling that involves the breakdown and reformation of bone tissue, which is regulated by a variety of hormones and other signaling molecules. Bone health is a critical aspect of overall health and well being, and it is affected by a range of factors including genetics, nutrition, physical activity, and age. Osteoporosis is a condition that occurs when bones become weakened and more susceptible to fractures, and it is a major public health issue that affects millions of people worldwide. In this chapter, we will discuss the structure and function of bones, as well as the causes and consequences of osteoporosis.

The Structure and Function of Bones:
Bones are composed of a variety of materials, including collagen fibers, calcium, and other minerals. These materials combine to form a complex matrix that provides both strength and flexibility to bone tissue. There are two main types of bone tissue: cortical bone and trabecular bone. Cortical

bone is the dense, outer layer of bone that forms the majority of the skeletal system, while trabecular bone is the more porous, inner layer that provides support and helps to distribute loads across the skeleton.

Bones have several important functions in the body. Perhaps the most obvious is their role in supporting and protecting the body's internal organs and tissues. The skeleton also plays a critical role in mobility, enabling movement through the action of muscles and tendons that attach to bones. Additionally, bones serve as a reservoir for important minerals such as calcium, which is critical for a range of physiological processes including muscle contraction and nerve function.

The Remodeling Process:

Bone is a dynamic tissue that undergoes constant remodeling in response to a variety of signals. The process of bone remodeling involves the breakdown and reformation of bone tissue, which is regulated by a variety of hormones and other signaling molecules. There are two types of cells involved in bone remodeling: osteoclasts and osteoblasts. Osteoclasts are specialized cells that break down old bone tissue, while osteoblasts are responsible for forming new bone tissue.

The remodeling process is tightly regulated by a variety of hormones and other signaling molecules. Perhaps the most important of these is parathyroid hormone (PTH), which is produced by the parathyroid gland and acts to increase calcium levels in the blood. PTH stimulates osteoclasts to break down old bone tissue, releasing calcium into the bloodstream. This, in turn, stimulates the production of new bone tissue by osteoblasts.

Other hormones and signaling molecules involved in bone remodeling include vitamin D, estrogen, testosterone, and calcitonin. Vitamin D is critical for the absorption of calcium from the diet and is therefore essential for bone health. Estrogen and testosterone are also important regulators of bone remodeling, with low levels of these hormones being associated with increased risk of osteoporosis. Calcitonin is produced by the thyroid gland and acts to decrease calcium levels in the blood, inhibiting the activity of osteoclasts.

Definition and causes of osteoporosis

Osteoporosis is a medical condition characterized by the thinning and weakening of bones, which makes them brittle and more prone to fractures. This disease is common in older adults, particularly women, and can lead to significant pain, disability, and even mortality. Osteoporosis is often called the "silent disease" because it typically does not cause any noticeable symptoms until a fracture occurs. In this article, we will define osteoporosis, discuss its causes, and explore its risk factors, diagnosis, and treatment.

Definition of Osteoporosis

Osteoporosis is a medical condition that affects the bones, making them weaker and more fragile. This can increase the risk of fractures, particularly in the hip, spine, and wrist. Osteoporosis is a progressive disease, meaning that it worsens over time, and it can be a significant source of pain, disability, and loss of independence.

Osteoporosis is caused by an imbalance between the processes that build new bone tissue and those that break down old bone tissue. Normally, the body constantly produces new bone tissue to replace old or damaged bone tissue. However, as we age, this process becomes less efficient, leading to a gradual loss of bone mass and density. In some people, this process can become accelerated, leading to the development of osteoporosis.

Causes of Osteoporosis

The primary cause of osteoporosis is a decrease in bone mass and density, which can be caused by a variety of factors. The most common causes of osteoporosis include:

Age: As we age, our bones naturally become less dense and more fragile, increasing the risk of osteoporosis.

Hormonal changes: Changes in hormones, particularly a decrease in estrogen levels in women after menopause, can contribute to the development of osteoporosis.

Genetics: Some people are genetically predisposed to developing osteoporosis, especially those with a family history of the disease.

Medications: Certain medications, such as glucocorticoids and some anticonvulsants, can increase the risk of osteoporosis.

Lifestyle factors: Certain lifestyle factors can also contribute to the development of osteoporosis, such as a diet low in calcium and vitamin D, smoking, excessive alcohol consumption, and a sedentary lifestyle.

Risk Factors for Osteoporosis

There are several factors that can increase a person's risk of developing osteoporosis. Some of the most common risk factors include:

Age: The risk of developing osteoporosis increases with age, particularly after the age of 50.

Gender: Women are more likely than men to develop osteoporosis, primarily because of the decrease in estrogen levels that occurs after menopause.

Genetics: A family history of osteoporosis can increase the risk of developing the disease.

Race: People of Caucasian and Asian descent are more likely to develop osteoporosis than those of other races.

Body weight: People who are underweight or have a small body frame are at greater risk of developing osteoporosis.

Hormonal factors: Women who experience early menopause or have their ovaries removed are at greater risk of developing osteoporosis.

Medications: Certain medications, such as glucocorticoids and some anticonvulsants, can increase the risk of osteoporosis.

Lifestyle factors: Smoking, excessive alcohol consumption, and a sedentary lifestyle can increase the risk of osteoporosis.

Diagnosis of Osteoporosis

Osteoporosis can be diagnosed through a combination of medical history, physical examination, and diagnostic tests. The most common tests used to diagnose osteoporosis include:

Bone density testing: This test uses a special X-ray called a DXA scan to measure bone density in the hip and spine. This test can help to determine the presence and severity of osteoporosis.

Blood tests: Blood tests can help to identify any underlying conditions that may be contributing to the development of osteoporosis, such as hyperthyroidism or vitamin D deficiency.

Urine tests: Urine tests can help to identify any abnormalities in the body's mineral metabolism that may be contributing to the development of osteoporosis.

Spine imaging: Imaging tests such as X-rays or CT scans can help to identify any fractures or abnormalities in the spine that may be related to osteoporosis.

Treatment of Osteoporosis

The treatment of osteoporosis typically involves a combination of lifestyle modifications, medications, and sometimes surgery. The goals of treatment are to slow or stop the progression of the disease, prevent fractures, and improve quality of life.

Lifestyle modifications: Lifestyle modifications such as regular exercise, a diet high in calcium and vitamin D, and avoidance of smoking and excessive alcohol consumption can help to slow the progression of osteoporosis and reduce the risk of fractures.

Medications: Medications such as bisphosphonates, hormone replacement therapy, and selective estrogen receptor modulators (SERMs) can help to slow bone loss and reduce the risk of fractures in people with osteoporosis.

Surgery: In severe cases of osteoporosis, surgery may be necessary to repair or stabilize fractures. Procedures such as kyphoplasty or vertebroplasty can help to relieve pain and improve mobility in people with spinal fractures.

CHAPTER 1

Osteoporosis is a common and potentially debilitating condition characterized by the thinning and weakening of bones. It can lead to significant pain, disability, and loss of independence, particularly in older adults. The primary cause of osteoporosis is a decrease in bone mass and density, which can be caused by a variety of factors such as age, hormonal changes, genetics, medications, and lifestyle factors. The diagnosis of osteoporosis typically involves a combination of medical history, physical examination, and diagnostic tests such as bone density testing and imaging. The treatment of osteoporosis typically involves a combination of lifestyle modifications, medications, and sometimes surgery, with the goals of slowing or stopping the progression of the disease, preventing fractures, and improving quality of life.

Signs and symptoms of osteoporosis

Osteoporosis is a skeletal disorder that results in decreased bone density and an increased risk of fractures. The condition is common, affecting millions of people worldwide, and is more prevalent among women, especially post-menopausal women. Osteoporosis typically develops gradually and without symptoms, so it may be difficult to detect in its early stages. However, as the condition progresses, certain signs and symptoms may become apparent. In this article, we will discuss the signs and symptoms of osteoporosis in detail.

Back pain: One of the most common symptoms of osteoporosis is back pain. This can occur due to fractures or compression of the vertebrae in the spine, which can cause the bones to collapse or become wedge-shaped. The pain is typically localized and may be aggravated by movement, especially bending or twisting.

Loss of height: Osteoporosis can cause a loss of height, as the bones in the spine become compressed or collapse. This can result in a stooped or hunched posture, which can further exacerbate back pain.

Fractures: Osteoporosis increases the risk of fractures, particularly in the hip, wrist, and spine. Fractures may occur as a result of minor falls or trauma that would not normally cause a fracture in someone without osteoporosis. Hip fractures, in particular, can be serious and may require surgery and a prolonged period of rehabilitation.

Weak and brittle nails: People with osteoporosis may have weak and brittle nails, which may break or split easily. This can be due to a lack of nutrients, such as calcium and vitamin D, which are important for nail health and bone strength.

Dental problems: Osteoporosis can affect dental health, as the jawbone is also made up of bone tissue. People with osteoporosis may experience tooth loss, gum disease, or difficulty with dentures.

Joint pain: Osteoporosis can cause joint pain, especially in the wrists, hips, and knees. This can be due to stress fractures or bone spurs that develop as a result of the condition.

Muscle weakness: Osteoporosis can lead to muscle weakness, which can make it difficult to perform everyday tasks. This can further increase the risk of falls and fractures.

Poor posture: Osteoporosis can cause poor posture, as the bones in the spine become compressed or collapse. This can result in a stooped or hunched posture, which can further exacerbate back pain.

Kyphosis: Kyphosis is a condition in which the spine becomes excessively curved, resulting in a hunchbacked appearance. This can occur in people with osteoporosis due to compression fractures of the vertebrae in the spine.

Loss of mobility: Osteoporosis can lead to a loss of mobility, as fractures and joint pain can make it difficult to move around. This can result in a decreased quality of life and an increased risk of further health complications.

Fatigue: People with osteoporosis may experience fatigue, which can be due to a lack of physical activity or anemia (a condition in which there are not enough red blood cells to carry oxygen throughout the body).

Depression: Osteoporosis can also contribute to depression, as the condition can lead to a loss of mobility and independence, as well as chronic pain.

Osteoporosis is a common condition that can lead to a range of symptoms, including back pain, loss of height, fractures, weak and brittle nails, dental problems, joint pain, muscle weakness, poor posture, kyphosis, loss of mobility, fatigue, and depression. If you are experiencing any of these symptoms, it is important to consult a healthcare provider for a proper diagnosis and treatment plan. Early detection and management of osteoporosis can help to prevent or slow down the progression of the condition and reduce the risk of fractures and other complications.

Risk factors for developing osteoporosis

There are several risk factors that can increase the likelihood of developing osteoporosis. These risk factors can be grouped into modifiable and non-modifiable factors.

Non Modifiable factors:

Age: As you get older, your risk of developing osteoporosis increases. This is because bones tend to become weaker and less dense as you age.

Gender: Women are more likely to develop osteoporosis than men. This is because women generally have lower bone density than men, and they also experience a rapid loss of bone mass after menopause due to the decrease in estrogen levels.

Genetics: Osteoporosis tends to run in families, so if you have a parent or sibling with the condition, you may be more likely to develop it yourself.

Body size: People who have a small body frame or are thin may be at greater risk for osteoporosis because they have less bone mass to begin with.

Ethnicity: Caucasian and Asian women are more likely to develop osteoporosis than women of other ethnicities.

Previous fractures: If you have already had a fracture due to osteoporosis, you are at increased risk for future fractures.

It is important to be aware of these non-modifiable risk factors for osteoporosis, as well as the modifiable risk factors that you can control, such as diet, exercise, and lifestyle habits, in order to take steps to prevent or manage the condition.

Modifiable factors:

CHAPTER 1

Modifiable risk factors for osteoporosis are those that you can control or change. By addressing these factors, you may be able to reduce your risk of developing osteoporosis or slow down its progression. Here are some of the modifiable risk factors:

Diet: A diet that is low in calcium and vitamin D can contribute to bone loss and increase the risk of osteoporosis. You can help prevent or manage osteoporosis by eating a diet rich in calcium and vitamin D. Good sources of calcium include dairy products, leafy green vegetables, and fortified foods such as orange juice and cereals. Vitamin D can be obtained from sunlight exposure, fatty fish, and fortified foods.

Physical activity: Regular exercise, especially weight-bearing and resistance exercises, can help improve bone density and reduce the risk of osteoporosis. Examples of weight-bearing exercises include walking, jogging, hiking, and dancing. Resistance exercises include weightlifting and other exercises that use resistance bands or weights.

Smoking: Smoking has been linked to a higher risk of osteoporosis, as it can reduce bone density and decrease the amount of calcium absorbed by the body. Quitting smoking can help reduce this risk.

Alcohol consumption: Excessive alcohol consumption can interfere with calcium absorption and increase the risk of bone loss and fractures. Limiting alcohol intake can help reduce the risk of osteoporosis.

Medications: Certain medications, such as glucocorticoids and some anti-convulsants, can increase the risk of osteoporosis. If you are taking these medications, talk to your healthcare provider about ways to manage your bone health.

Hormone levels: Women who experience early menopause or have low estrogen levels are at increased risk of osteoporosis. Hormone replacement therapy (HRT) may be recommended to help reduce this risk.

Body weight: Being underweight or losing weight rapidly can increase the risk of osteoporosis. Maintaining a healthy body weight through a balanced diet and regular exercise can help protect your bones.

By addressing these modifiable risk factors, you can help prevent or manage osteoporosis and maintain strong and healthy bones.

Complications of osteoporosis

Some of the complications that can arise from osteoporosis include:

Fractures: Osteoporosis is a leading cause of fractures, especially in the hip, spine, and wrist. These fractures can be very painful and can severely impact quality of life.

Decreased mobility and independence: Fractures caused by osteoporosis can limit mobility and reduce independence, as people may no longer be able to perform daily tasks such as walking, climbing stairs, or even getting out of bed.

Chronic pain: Fractures caused by osteoporosis can lead to chronic pain that may persist long after the fracture has healed.

Spinal deformity: Osteoporosis can cause vertebrae in the spine to collapse or become compressed, leading to a stooped or hunched posture known as kyphosis.

Reduced lung function: Severe kyphosis can compress the lungs and reduce lung function, leading to breathing difficulties.

Reduced quality of life: The pain and disability caused by osteoporosis can lead to depression, social isolation, and reduced quality of life.

Increased mortality: Fractures caused by osteoporosis can lead to increased mortality, especially in older adults.

Chapter 2

Why Exercise is Crucial for Osteoporosis?:

How exercise can help prevent and manage osteoporosis

Before we dive into the benefits of exercise for osteoporosis, it is important to understand what happens to bones as we age. Bone is a living tissue that is constantly being broken down and replaced by new bone tissue. As we age, the rate of bone breakdown starts to exceed the rate of bone formation, leading to a loss of bone density and mass. This loss of bone density and mass can make bones weaker and more susceptible to fractures.

Exercise is crucial for osteoporosis because it helps to maintain and improve bone density and mass. When we engage in weight-bearing exercise, such as walking, jogging, or weightlifting, our bones are subjected to forces that stimulate the formation of new bone tissue. This process is called bone remodeling, and it is essential for maintaining bone strength and density.

Increases bone density: Weight-bearing exercise, such as walking, running, dancing, and weightlifting, can help increase bone density, which in turn can reduce the risk of osteoporosis.

Strengthens muscles: Exercise can help strengthen the muscles surrounding the bones, which can reduce the risk of falls and fractures. Stronger muscles also help to improve balance and stability.

Improves balance and coordination: Exercise can improve balance and coordination, which can reduce the risk of falls and fractures.

Enhances flexibility: Exercise can help improve flexibility, which can reduce the risk of falls and fractures. Improved flexibility can also help to reduce the risk of muscle strains and joint pain.

Reduces inflammation: Exercise has anti-inflammatory effects that can help reduce inflammation in the body, which is a risk factor for osteoporosis.

Helps manage weight: Exercise can help manage weight, which can reduce the risk of osteoporosis. Being overweight can increase the risk of osteoporosis due to the increased strain on the bones.

It's important to note that exercise alone may not be enough to prevent or manage osteoporosis. Other lifestyle factors, such as a healthy diet and not smoking, which we shall be discussing properly below are also important. It's also important to speak with your doctor before beginning any exercise program, especially if you have been diagnosed with osteoporosis or have a history of fractures.

Benefits of exercise for bone health

Certainly. Exercise has numerous benefits for bone health, and it is crucial to engage in regular physical activity to maintain and improve bone health. In this essay, we will discuss the benefits of exercise for bone health, including the mechanisms behind these benefits, the types of exercise that are most effective, and the recommended guidelines for exercise for bone health.

Benefits of Exercise for Bone Health:
Exercise has been shown to have numerous benefits for bone health, including increasing bone density, reducing the risk of fractures, and improving overall bone strength. These benefits are particularly important for older adults who are at a higher risk of developing osteoporosis and other bone-related conditions.

Increased Bone Density:
Bone density refers to the amount of bone tissue in a certain area of the bone. Low bone density is a significant risk factor for fractures, particularly in older adults. Exercise has been shown to increase bone density by stimulating bone growth and strengthening the existing bone tissue. High-impact activities such as running, jumping, and weightlifting have been shown to be particularly effective in increasing bone density.

Reduced Risk of Fractures:
Regular exercise can help reduce the risk of fractures by increasing bone density and improving overall bone strength. Exercise also helps improve balance and coordination, which can help prevent falls, a common cause of fractures in older adults.

Improved Bone Strength:

Exercise can improve bone strength by increasing the size and density of the bone, making it more resistant to fracture. This is particularly important in older adults who may experience a decline in bone strength due to age-related changes in bone physiology.

Reduced Risk of Falls:

Exercise can improve balance and coordination, which can help reduce the risk of falls and associated fractures. By engaging in activities that challenge balance and proprioception, such as yoga or tai chi, older adults can improve their ability to maintain balance and prevent falls.

Reduced Risk of Chronic Disease:

Regular exercise has been shown to reduce the risk of chronic diseases such as heart disease, type 2 diabetes, and certain types of cancer. These diseases have been linked to bone loss and an increased risk of fractures, so reducing the risk of these conditions through exercise can have a positive impact on bone health.

Improved Quality of Life:

Maintaining good bone health can have a significant impact on an individual's quality of life. By reducing the risk of fractures and maintaining mobility and independence, exercise can help individuals maintain an active and fulfilling lifestyle as they age. Additionally, the social and psychological benefits of exercise can also contribute to improved overall well-being.

Mechanisms Behind the Benefits of Exercise for Bone Health

The benefits of exercise for bone health are due to several mechanisms. First, exercise stimulates bone growth by putting stress on the bone tissue. This stress stimulates the bone cells to produce more bone tissue, resulting in increased bone density. Second, exercise helps improve bone quality by increasing the size and density of the bone tissue. This makes the bone stronger and more resistant to fracture. Finally, exercise can help improve balance and coordination, which can help prevent falls, a common cause of fractures in older adults.

Types of exercises recommended for osteoporosis

The following types of exercises are recommended for people with osteoporosis:

Weight-bearing exercises: These are exercises that require you to support your own body weight, such as walking, hiking, dancing, and stair climbing. These exercises can help to strengthen bones and reduce the risk of fractures.

Resistance exercises: These are exercises that involve lifting weights or using resistance bands to strengthen muscles and bones. Examples include lifting weights, doing squats, and using resistance bands.

Balance exercises: These are exercises that improve balance and coordination, reducing the risk of falls. Examples include standing on one foot, heel-to-toe walking, and Tai Chi.

Flexibility exercises: These are exercises that stretch muscles and improve joint mobility. Examples include yoga, Pilates, and stretching exercises.

Cycling: Cycling is a low-impact aerobic exercise that can help to strengthen leg muscles and improve cardiovascular fitness. Cycling on a stationary bike or outdoors can be a good option for people with osteoporosis who may be at risk for falls or fractures.

Swimming: Swimming is another low-impact aerobic exercise that can help to strengthen muscles and bones without putting stress on the joints. Swimming can also be a good option for people with osteoporosis who may have joint pain or limited mobility.

Weighted Squats: Weighted squats can help to strengthen the lower body, including the hips, thighs, and glutes. Stand with your feet shoulder-width apart, holding a dumbbell or kettlebell in each hand. Lower into a squat position, keeping your back straight and your knees behind your toes. Then, return to the starting position and repeat for several reps. Gradually increase the weight as you become stronger. It's important to use proper form and start with a weight that is comfortable for you.

Note that all these exercises listed above are just for formality purposes, we are going to explain elaborately on them in the subsequent topics.

How often and how much exercise is necessary for osteoporosis?

Regular exercise is an essential component of the management of osteoporosis. It can help prevent further bone loss and reduce the risk of fractures. The frequency and intensity of exercise required for osteoporosis may vary depending on factors such as age, gender, overall health, and the severity of the condition. However, the following are some general guidelines:

Frequency: Engage in weight-bearing exercise at least three to four times a week. Weight-bearing exercise includes activities such as walking, jogging, dancing, and aerobics.

Duration: Aim for at least 30 minutes of weight-bearing exercise per session.

Intensity: Choose exercises that challenge the bones and muscles, but are still safe and appropriate for your fitness level. Examples include brisk walking, hiking, stair climbing, and weightlifting.

Variety: Incorporate a variety of exercises to target different muscle groups and prevent boredom.

Consult with a healthcare professional: Before starting any exercise program, it is important to consult with a healthcare professional to determine what exercises are safe and appropriate for you.

It's important to note that the intensity of the exercise and the level of impact should be appropriate for an individual's current fitness level and bone density. Activities that are too strenuous or high-impact can increase the risk of falls and fractures, especially in those with severe osteoporosis. Therefore, it's recommended that individuals with osteoporosis work with a qualified healthcare provider or certified exercise specialist to design a safe and effective exercise program.

safety tips for your exercises and exercises you should avoid

people with osteoporosis should exercise with caution and follow some safety tips to avoid injury, we'll look at some of the safety tips for exercise and exercises you should avoid when dealing with osteoporosis.

Safety Tips for Exercise

Consult with Your Doctor Before Starting an Exercise Program
   It's essential to talk to your doctor before starting any exercise program, especially if you have osteoporosis. Your doctor can help you determine the

types of exercise that are appropriate for your current health status and bone density. They can also help you set realistic goals and tailor a program that meets your individual needs.

Choose Safe Activities

The type of exercise you choose can significantly impact your bone health. Weight-bearing and resistance exercises are the most effective for maintaining and improving bone density. Examples of weight-bearing exercises include walking, hiking, jogging, dancing, stair climbing, and elliptical training. Resistance exercises such as weightlifting, bodyweight exercises, or resistance band training, target the muscles and bones in the upper and lower body, which can help to maintain bone mass and reduce the risk of fractures. On the other hand, high-impact exercises such as running and jumping can be dangerous for people with osteoporosis, as they increase the risk of fractures.

Start Slow and Gradually Increase Intensity

It's crucial to start slowly and gradually increase the intensity of your exercise program. This approach can help you avoid injury and build strength over time. Start with low-impact activities and resistance exercises, and then gradually increase the duration and intensity of your workouts as you get stronger. Aim for at least 30 minutes of moderate-intensity exercise most days of the week.

Use Proper Form and Technique

Using proper form and technique when exercising is crucial to avoid injury and improve the effectiveness of your exercises. Consider working with a certified exercise specialist or physical therapist who can teach you proper form and technique. They can also help you modify exercises to meet your individual needs.

Wear Proper Footwear

Wearing proper footwear when exercising is essential to prevent falls and injuries. Choose shoes that are comfortable, provide good support, and have a non-slip sole. Avoid wearing shoes with high heels or narrow soles that can increase the risk of falls.

Use Safety Equipment

When performing resistance exercises, use safety equipment such as weight belts, lifting gloves, and straps. These tools can help you maintain proper form and protect your hands and wrists from injury.

Stay Hydrated

Staying hydrated is crucial when exercising, especially if you have osteoporosis. Drink plenty of water before, during, and after exercise to prevent dehydration and maintain proper fluid balance in your body.

Exercises You Should Avoid

High-Impact Exercises

High-impact exercises such as running, jumping, and high-intensity interval training can be dangerous for people with osteoporosis. These exercises can increase the risk of fractures and should be avoided or performed with caution.

Twisting Exercises

Twisting exercises such as golf swings, tennis serves, and trunk rotations can put stress on the spine and increase the risk of vertebral fractures. Consider modifying these exercises or avoiding them altogether.

Exercises That Involve Bending Forward

Exercises that involve bending forward can also increase the risk of vertebral fractures. Avoid exercises such as sit-ups, crunches, and toe touches, which can put undue stress on the spine. Instead, focus on exercises that strengthen the core muscles without bending forward, such as planks, bridges, and pelvic tilts.

Exercises with Heavy Weights

While resistance exercises are essential for maintaining bone density, exercises with heavy weights can put too much stress on the bones and increase the risk of fractures. Instead, focus on light to moderate weights and perform more repetitions to achieve the desired level of intensity.

Exercises that Require Twisting and Bending Simultaneously

Exercises that require twisting and bending simultaneously, such as combining a side bend with a twisting motion, can also increase the risk of fractures. Instead, choose exercises that involve one motion at a time, such as a simple side bend or a twisting motion without bending.

Exercises that Involve Rapid Movements

Exercises that involve rapid movements or sudden changes in direction, such as plyometric exercises, can also increase the risk of fractures. Instead, choose exercises that involve slow and controlled movements to reduce the risk of injury.

Exercises that Involve Unsupported Forward Bends

Exercises that involve unsupported forward bends, such as toe touches, can put undue stress on the spine and increase the risk of vertebral fractures. Instead, choose exercises that involve a supported forward bend, such as seated forward bends with the support of a block or a bolster.

Regular exercise is an essential component of bone health for people with osteoporosis. However, it's crucial to exercise with caution and follow safety tips to avoid injury. Choosing safe activities, starting slow, using proper form, and avoiding high-impact exercises can help reduce the risk of fractures and improve bone density. On the other hand, exercises that involve twisting, bending forward, heavy weights, rapid movements, unsupported forward bends, and combinations of these movements should be avoided or modified to reduce the risk of injury. Remember to consult with your doctor or a certified exercise specialist before starting any exercise program and tailor your program to meet your individual needs. With proper care and attention, exercise can be a safe and effective way to maintain bone health and reduce the risk of fractures for people with osteoporosis.

There are other lifestyle factors that can help to prevent and manage osteoporosis. These include:

Nutrition: Eating a balanced diet that is rich in calcium and vitamin D is important for bone health. Calcium is essential for building and maintaining strong bones, while vitamin D helps the body to absorb calcium. Good sources of calcium include dairy products, leafy green vegetables, and fortified foods such as cereals and orange juice. Good sources of vitamin D include fatty fish, egg yolks, and fortified foods such as milk and cereal.

Smoking cessation: Smoking has been linked to a decrease in bone density and an increased risk of fractures. Quitting smoking can help to improve bone health and reduce the risk of fractures.

Limiting alcohol consumption: Excessive alcohol consumption can also have a negative impact on bone health. Limiting alcohol consumption can help to prevent bone loss and reduce the risk of fractures.

3

Chapter 3

Building a Strong Foundation:

When it comes to building a strong foundation for people with osteoporosis, the focus should be on exercises that improve balance, posture, and strength, as well as those that promote bone density.

Building a strong foundation for people with osteoporosis involves several key steps:

Nutrition: Eating a well-balanced diet rich in calcium, vitamin D, and other nutrients that support bone health is essential for people with osteoporosis. Calcium is particularly important for building and maintaining strong bones. Good sources of calcium include dairy products, leafy green vegetables, and fortified foods. Vitamin D is also essential for bone health, as it helps the body absorb calcium. Good sources of vitamin D include fatty fish, egg yolks, and fortified foods.

Lifestyle modifications: People with osteoporosis should avoid smoking and excessive alcohol consumption, as both can increase the risk of bone loss and fractures. Additionally, people with osteoporosis should be careful when participating in activities that could increase the risk of falls, such as climbing ladders, standing on chairs or stools, and walking on uneven surfaces.

Medications: Depending on the severity of the osteoporosis, a healthcare provider may prescribe medication to help slow down bone loss and reduce the risk of fractures. These medications may include bisphosphonates, hormone replacement therapy, or other bone-building drugs.

Fall prevention: Finally, people with osteoporosis should take steps to prevent falls. This can include modifying the home environment by removing tripping hazards, installing grab bars and handrails, and using non-slip mats in the bathroom. Additionally, people with osteoporosis should wear appropriate footwear and use assistive devices such as canes or walkers if necessary.

Regular check-ups: Regular check-ups with a healthcare provider are important for people with osteoporosis. They can monitor bone density levels and make adjustments to the treatment plan as needed. Additionally, healthcare providers can provide guidance on lifestyle modifications, fall prevention, and other strategies for managing osteoporosis.

Strength and balance training: While I won't go into specific exercises, strength and balance training can be very helpful for people with osteoporosis. Strengthening the muscles can help support the bones and reduce the risk of fractures, while balance training can help prevent falls. It's important to work with a healthcare provider or certified fitness professional to develop a safe and effective exercise plan.

Adequate rest: Adequate rest and sleep are important for overall health, including bone health. Getting enough sleep can help the body repair and regenerate bone tissue, while inadequate sleep can interfere with the body's ability to do so.

Stress management: Chronic stress can have negative effects on bone health. Practicing stress management techniques such as meditation, yoga, or deep breathing can help reduce stress levels and promote overall health.

Social support: Living with osteoporosis can be challenging, and having a strong support network can be helpful. Friends, family members, support groups, or online forums can provide emotional support and practical advice for managing osteoporosis

Assessing your current fitness level

Assessing your current fitness level is an important first step in developing an effective exercise program. Here are some ways to assess your fitness level:

Resting heart rate: Your resting heart rate is the number of times your heart beats per minute while you are at rest. A lower resting heart rate is generally an indicator of good cardiovascular fitness. To measure your resting heart rate, sit quietly for a few minutes and then check your pulse at your wrist or neck. Count the number of beats for 60 seconds.

Blood pressure: Blood pressure is a measure of the force of blood against the walls of your arteries. High blood pressure is a risk factor for heart disease and other health problems. You can have your blood pressure measured at a healthcare provider's office, or you can purchase a home blood pressure monitor.

Body composition: Body composition refers to the ratio of fat to lean mass in your body. You can measure your body composition using various methods, including skinfold calipers, bioelectrical impedance analysis, or dual-energy x-ray absorptiometry (DXA).

Flexibility: Flexibility refers to the range of motion in your joints. Good flexibility can help prevent injury and improve overall mobility. You can measure your flexibility using various tests, including the sit-and-reach test and the shoulder flexibility test.

Strength: Strength refers to the amount of force your muscles can generate. You can measure your strength using various tests, including the one-repetition maximum (1RM) test and the hand grip strength test.

Endurance: Endurance refers to your ability to sustain physical activity for an extended period of time. You can measure your endurance using various tests, including the six-minute walk test and the VO2max test.

Once you have assessed your fitness level, you can use this information to develop an exercise program that is tailored to your needs and abilities. A healthcare provider or certified fitness professional can help you develop a safe and effective exercise plan.

Balance: Good balance is important for preventing falls, especially as we age. You can assess your balance using various tests, including the one-leg stand test and the tandem walk test.

Coordination: Coordination refers to your ability to perform complex movements efficiently and accurately. You can assess your coordination using various tests, including the finger-to-nose test and the heel-to-toe walk test.

Reaction time: Reaction time refers to how quickly you can respond to a stimulus. You can assess your reaction time using various tests, including the ruler drop test and the computer-based reaction time test.

Agility: Agility refers to your ability to change direction quickly and efficiently. You can assess your agility using various tests, including the agility run test and the T-test.

Bear it in mind that no single test can provide a complete picture of your fitness level. Instead, it's best to use a combination of tests to assess various aspects of your fitness. Also, it's important to interpret the results of your fitness tests in the context of your overall health and lifestyle. A healthcare provider or certified fitness professional can help you interpret your results and develop an appropriate exercise program based on your goals and abilities.

Developing a safe and effective exercise plan

Developing a safe and effective exercise plan is essential for improving fitness and reducing the risk of injury. Here are some tips for developing an exercise plan:

Set realistic goals: Setting realistic goals can help keep you motivated and focused. Be specific about what you want to achieve and give yourself a timeline for reaching your goals.

Choose activities you enjoy: Choosing activities that you enjoy can help make exercise more enjoyable and sustainable. Consider activities such as swimming, cycling, dancing, or walking.

Gradually increase intensity and duration: Gradually increasing the intensity and duration of your workouts can help prevent injury and improve fitness. Start with low-intensity workouts and gradually increase the intensity and duration over time.

Incorporate a variety of exercises: Incorporating a variety of exercises can help prevent boredom and challenge different muscle groups. Consider including aerobic exercise, strength training, and flexibility exercises in your workout routine.

Warm up and cool down: Warming up and cooling down can help prevent injury and improve performance. Start each workout with a few minutes of low-intensity exercise, such as walking or jogging, and end each workout with a few minutes of stretching.

Listen to your body: Pay attention to how your body feels during and after exercise. If you experience pain or discomfort, modify your workout or stop exercising altogether. It's important to listen to your body and not push yourself too hard.

Seek guidance from a healthcare provider or certified fitness professional: A healthcare provider or certified fitness professional can help you develop a safe and effective exercise plan based on your health status, fitness level, and goals. They can also provide guidance on proper exercise technique and modifications for any physical limitations or medical conditions.

Remember, the most important aspect of any exercise plan is consistency. Aim to exercise regularly, ideally at least three to five times per week, and gradually increase the intensity and duration of your workouts over time.

Starting slowly and gradually increasing intensity.

Starting slowly and gradually increasing intensity is a key component of developing a safe and effective exercise plan for people with osteoporosis. This approach allows the individual's body to adjust to the new exercise routine and helps prevent injury. Here are some tips to help with starting slowly and gradually increasing intensity:

Start with low-impact exercises: Low-impact exercises such as walking, swimming, and cycling are great options for starting an exercise program. These exercises are gentle on the joints and can be modified to suit the individual's fitness level.

Begin with short sessions: Start with short exercise sessions, such as 10-15 minutes, and gradually increase the duration as the individual's fitness level improves.

Increase intensity gradually: Once the individual is comfortable with the exercise routine, gradually increase the intensity by adding more resistance, increasing the speed or incline, or adding more repetitions.

Take rest days: Rest days are important for allowing the body to recover and preventing injury. Aim for at least one or two rest days per week.

Listen to the body: Pay attention to how the body feels during and after exercise. If there is pain or discomfort, reduce the intensity or stop the exercise altogether.

Consider working with a personal trainer or physical therapist: A personal trainer or physical therapist can help create an exercise plan that is tailored to the individual's needs and limitations, and can provide guidance on how to safely increase intensity over time.

Remember that exercise is important for maintaining bone health and overall well-being, but it's important to start slowly and gradually increase intensity to prevent injury and ensure a safe and effective exercise program.

Incorporate variety: Incorporating a variety of exercises can help prevent boredom and improve overall fitness. Try different types of exercises, such as strength training, balance exercises, and flexibility exercises.

Use proper form: Using proper form during exercise can help prevent injury and ensure the exercise is effective. Consider working with a personal trainer or physical therapist to learn proper form for each exercise.

Consider equipment and modifications: Some exercises may require equipment or modifications to make them safe and effective for people with osteoporosis. For example, using a stability ball or resistance bands can add variety and challenge to an exercise routine. Be sure to use equipment and modifications properly to avoid injury.

Be patient: Improvements in bone density and overall fitness take time, so it's important to be patient and consistent with the exercise program. Celebrate small successes along the way and keep a positive attitude to stay motivated.

Finding support and guidance for your exercise routine

Finding support and guidance for your exercise routine can help you stay motivated, ensure that you are performing exercises safely and effectively, and provide a sense of accountability. Here are some ways to find support and guidance for your exercise routine:

Work with a personal trainer or physical therapist: A personal trainer or physical therapist can provide guidance on creating an exercise plan that is tailored to your individual needs and limitations. They can also teach you proper form and technique for each exercise and help you track your progress.

Join a fitness class or group: Joining a fitness class or group can provide a sense of community and support. Look for classes specifically designed for people with osteoporosis, such as low-impact aerobics, yoga, or Pilates.

Use online resources: There are many online resources available for people with osteoporosis, such as exercise videos, forums, and support groups. Look for reputable sources, such as the National Osteoporosis Foundation or the American College of Sports Medicine.

Seek support from friends and family: Share your exercise goals and progress with friends and family members. They can provide encouragement and support along the way.

Consider a wearable fitness tracker: A wearable fitness tracker can help you track your progress and provide motivation to stay active.

Consult with a healthcare provider: Consult with a healthcare provider, such as a doctor or physical therapist, for guidance on finding support and guidance for your exercise routine

Participate in community events: Participating in community events, such as charity walks or runs, can be a great way to get active while also supporting a cause. This can also provide a sense of community and motivation to stay active.

Incorporate exercise into daily activities: Incorporating exercise into daily activities can help make physical activity a habit. This can include taking the stairs instead of the elevator, walking or biking to work, or doing household chores that involve physical activity.

Use apps and technology: There are many apps and technology available that can help track progress and provide motivation, such as workout apps, pedometers, and heart rate monitors.

Find a workout buddy: Finding a workout buddy can provide motivation, accountability, and support. Consider finding a friend, family member, or colleague who shares your exercise goals.

Choose the methods that work best for you and stick with them to achieve your exercise goals!!!.

Chapter 4

Resistance Training:

Definition and benefits of resistance training:

Resistance training is a form of exercise that involves working against a resistance to improve muscular strength and endurance. This type of training can take many forms, including weightlifting, using resistance bands, or using one's body weight. The resistance used can be either external, such as weights or bands, or internal, such as using one's own body weight. The primary goal of resistance training is to increase the strength and endurance of the muscles being worked, which can lead to improved overall physical function and performance.

Benefits of Resistance Training for Osteoporosis Patients:

Resistance training has been shown to have numerous benefits for individuals with osteoporosis. Some of the most significant benefits include:

Increased Bone Density: Resistance training has been shown to increase bone density in individuals with osteoporosis. This is because the forces placed on the bones during resistance training stimulate bone growth, leading to an increase in bone density.

Reduced Risk of Fractures: Osteoporosis patients are at an increased risk of fractures due to their weakened bones. Resistance training can help reduce this risk by increasing bone density and improving overall bone health. Additionally, resistance training can improve balance and stability, which can help prevent falls, a leading cause of fractures in osteoporosis patients.

Improved Muscle Strength and Endurance: Resistance training can improve muscle strength and endurance, which can help improve overall physical function and performance in osteoporosis patients. This can lead to an improved ability to perform activities of daily living, such as walking, climbing stairs, and carrying groceries.

Improved Body Composition: Resistance training can help improve body composition by increasing muscle mass and reducing fat mass. This can lead to improved overall health and a reduced risk of chronic diseases such as diabetes and heart disease.

Improved Quality of Life: Resistance training has been shown to improve quality of life in individuals with osteoporosis. This is because resistance training can improve physical function, reduce pain, and improve overall mood and mental health.

CHAPTER 4

Incorporating Resistance Training into an Osteoporosis Treatment Plan:

Resistance training can be an effective component of an osteoporosis treatment plan. However, it is important to work with a healthcare professional to develop a safe and effective exercise program that is tailored to the individual's specific needs and abilities. Here are some guidelines for incorporating resistance training into an osteoporosis treatment plan:

Start Slowly: It is important to start slowly and gradually increase the intensity of the resistance training program. This can help prevent injury and allow the body to adapt to the new stresses being placed on it.

Use Proper Technique: It is important to use proper technique when performing resistance exercises to avoid injury and maximize the benefits of the exercise. This may involve working with a trainer or physical therapist to learn proper form.

Incorporate Weight-Bearing Exercises: Weight-bearing exercises, such as walking, jogging, or dancing, can be an effective form of resistance training for individuals with osteoporosis. These exercises place stress on the bones, which can help improve bone density and reduce the risk of fractures

Focus on Large Muscle Groups: Resistance training exercises that focus on large muscle groups, such as the legs, back, and chest, can provide the most significant benefits for osteoporosis patients. These exercises can help improve overall muscle strength and endurance, which can lead to improved physical function and performance.

Use Progressive Overload: Progressive overload is the principle of gradually increasing the intensity or volume of an exercise program over time. This can help ensure continued improvements in strength and bone density. However, it is important to progress slowly and avoid overloading the body too quickly.

Consider Resistance Bands or Bodyweight Exercises: For individuals who are unable to lift weights or use weight machines, resistance bands or bodyweight exercises can be an effective form of resistance training. These exercises can be modified to suit an individual's abilities and can be performed at home or in a gym.

Consider Safety Precautions: It is important to take safety precautions when performing resistance training exercises, particularly for individuals with osteoporosis. This may include using a spotter when lifting weights, wearing appropriate footwear, and avoiding exercises that place excessive stress on the spine.

Examples of resistance exercises:

Resistance exercises can be very beneficial for individuals with osteoporosis, as they help to build bone density and strength. Here are some examples of resistance exercises that can be helpful for individuals with osteoporosis:

Squats:

Squats are a great exercise for building lower body strength. Start with bodyweight squats and gradually add weights as your strength improves.

Lunges:

Lunges are another effective lower body exercise that can help to build strength in the legs and hips. Start with bodyweight lunges and gradually add weights as your strength improves.

Wall push-ups:

Wall push-ups are a good upper body exercise that can help to build strength in the chest, shoulders, and arms. Stand facing a wall with your hands flat against the wall at shoulder height, then push yourself away from the wall.

Seated rows:

Seated rows are a good exercise for building upper back and shoulder strength. Sit on a chair with your feet flat on the floor, then hold a resistance band or dumbbells and pull them towards your chest while keeping your elbows close to your sides.

Standing calf raises:

Standing calf raises are a good exercise for building calf strength. Stand on the edge of a step with your heels hanging off the edge, then rise up onto your toes and slowly lower yourself back down.

It's important to work with a qualified healthcare professional or physical therapist to develop a safe and effective resistance exercise program that is tailored to your individual needs and abilities.

Daily routine plan and time table for resistance exercises:

Daily routine plan and time table for squats:

Warm-up: It's important to warm up before you start your squat routine. This can include a few minutes of light cardio exercise, such as walking or cycling, followed by some dynamic stretching to get your muscles ready for the workout.

Set your goals: Decide on your goals for your squat routine. Are you looking to build strength or improve your endurance? How many sets and reps will you do? Setting goals can help you stay focused and motivated during your workout.

Squat routine:

- Set 1: 3-5 reps at 50% of your one-rep max (1RM), with a rest period of 60 seconds between sets.
- Set 2: 3-5 reps at 75% of your 1RM, with a rest period of 90 seconds between sets.
- Set 3: 3-5 reps at 85% of your 1RM, with a rest period of 120 seconds between sets.
- Set 4: 1-2 reps at 90% of your 1RM, with a rest period of 120 seconds between sets.
- Set 5: 1 rep at 95% of your 1RM, with a rest period of 120 seconds between sets.

Cool down: After your squat routine, it's important to cool down and stretch your muscles to prevent injury and reduce muscle soreness. Spend 5-10 minutes doing some light cardio exercise, such as walking or cycling, followed by some static stretching to help your muscles relax.

Rest and recovery: Allow your body time to rest and recover after your squat routine. Depending on your goals and fitness level, you may want to do this routine every other day or 2-3 times per week.

Remember, this is just a sample routine and may not be appropriate for everyone. Always consult with a qualified fitness professional before starting any new exercise routine, and listen to your body to avoid injury.

Daily routine plan and time table for lunges:

Warm-up: Start with a few minutes of light cardio exercise, such as jogging or cycling, to get your heart rate up and your muscles warm. Follow with some dynamic stretching, such as walking lunges, to prepare your body for the workout.

Set your goals: Decide on your goals for your lunge routine. Are you looking to build strength, improve your balance, or increase your endurance? How many sets and reps will you do? Setting goals can help you stay focused and motivated during your workout.

Lunge routine:

-
  - Set 1: 10-12 reps of forward lunges on each leg, with a rest period of 60 seconds between sets.
  - Set 2: 10-12 reps of lateral lunges on each leg, with a rest period of 60 seconds between sets.
  - Set 3: 10-12 reps of reverse lunges on each leg, with a rest period of 60 seconds between sets.

- Set 4: 10-12 reps of walking lunges, alternating legs, with a rest period of 60 seconds between sets.

Cool down: After your lunge routine, it's important to cool down and stretch your muscles to prevent injury and reduce muscle soreness. Spend 5-10 minutes doing some light cardio exercise, such as walking or cycling, followed by some static stretching to help your muscles relax.

Rest and recovery: Allow your body time to rest and recover after your lunge routine. Depending on your goals and fitness level, you may want to do this routine every other day or 2-3 times per week.

Daily routine plan and time table for wall push-ups:

Warm-up: Start with a few minutes of light cardio exercise, such as jogging or jumping jacks, to get your heart rate up and your muscles warm. Follow with some dynamic stretching to prepare your body for the workout.

Set your goals: Decide on your goals for your wall push-up routine. Are you looking to build strength in your chest, shoulders, and arms? How many sets and reps will you do? Setting goals can help you stay focused and motivated during your workout.

Wall push-up routine:

- Set 1: 10-12 reps of wall push-ups, with a rest period of 60 seconds between sets.
- Set 2: 10-12 reps of incline push-ups, using a bench or elevated surface, with a rest period of 60 seconds between sets.

- Set 3: 10-12 reps of decline push-ups, using a low bench or stairs, with a rest period of 60 seconds between sets.
- Set 4: 10-12 reps of diamond push-ups, with your hands close together in a diamond shape, with a rest period of 60 seconds between sets.

Cool down: After your wall push-up routine, it's important to cool down and stretch your muscles to prevent injury and reduce muscle soreness. Spend 5-10 minutes doing some light cardio exercise, such as walking or cycling, followed by some static stretching to help your muscles relax.

Rest and recovery: Allow your body time to rest and recover after your wall push-up routine. Depending on your goals and fitness level, you may want to do this routine every other day or 2-3 times per week.

Daily routine plan and time table for seated rows

Warm-up: Start with a few minutes of light cardio exercise, such as jogging or cycling, to get your heart rate up and your muscles warm. Follow with some dynamic stretching to prepare your body for the workout.

Set your goals: Decide on your goals for your seated row routine. Are you looking to build strength in your back, shoulders, and arms? How many sets and reps will you do? Setting goals can help you stay focused and motivated during your workout.

Seated row routine:

-
- Set 1: 10-12 reps of seated rows with a light weight, with a rest period of 60 seconds between sets.
- Set 2: 10-12 reps of seated rows with a moderate weight, with a rest period

of 60 seconds between sets.
- Set 3: 10-12 reps of seated rows with a heavy weight, with a rest period of 60 seconds between sets.
- Set 4: 10-12 reps of single arm seated rows, alternating arms, with a rest period of 60 seconds between sets.

Cool down: After your seated row routine, it's important to cool down and stretch your muscles to prevent injury and reduce muscle soreness. Spend 5-10 minutes doing some light cardio exercise, such as walking or cycling, followed by some static stretching to help your muscles relax.

Rest and recovery: Allow your body time to rest and recover after your seated row routine. Depending on your goals and fitness level, you may want to do this routine every other day or 2-3 times per week.

Daily routine plan and time table for Standing calf raises

Warm-up: Start with a few minutes of light cardio exercise, such as jogging or jumping jacks, to get your heart rate up and your muscles warm. Follow with some dynamic stretching to prepare your body for the workout.

Set your goals: Decide on your goals for your standing calf raise routine. Are you looking to build strength and size in your calf muscles? How many sets and reps will you do? Setting goals can help you stay focused and motivated during your workout.

Standing calf raise routine:

- Set 1: 12-15 reps of standing calf raises with both feet, with a rest period

of 60 seconds between sets.
- Set 2: 12-15 reps of standing calf raises with one foot, with a rest period of 60 seconds between sets. Repeat on the other foot.
- Set 3: 12-15 reps of standing calf raises with both feet, with a weight or resistance band, with a rest period of 60 seconds between sets.
- Set 4: 12-15 reps of standing calf raises with one foot, with a weight or resistance band, with a rest period of 60 seconds between sets. Repeat on the other foot.

Cool down: After your standing calf raise routine, it's important to cool down and stretch your muscles to prevent injury and reduce muscle soreness. Spend 5-10 minutes doing some light cardio exercise, such as walking or cycling, followed by some static stretching to help your muscles relax.

Rest and recovery: Allow your body time to rest and recover after your standing calf raise routine. Depending on your goals and fitness level, you may want to do this routine every other day or 2-3 times per week.

Safety precautions for resistance training:

Resistance training can be a safe and effective way to manage osteoporosis, but it's important to take certain safety precautions to prevent injury. Here are some safety precautions to consider when doing resistance training for osteoporosis:

Consult with a healthcare professional: Before beginning any resistance training program, consult with your healthcare professional to ensure that it's safe for you to do so.

Start slow and gradually increase the intensity: Begin with lighter weights or resistance bands and gradually increase the intensity over time. This will help prevent injury and allow your body to adjust to the new exercise.

Use proper technique: Proper technique is important to ensure that you're targeting the correct muscles and avoiding unnecessary strain on your joints. Consider working with a qualified fitness professional to learn proper technique.

Avoid high-impact exercises: High-impact exercises, such as jumping or running, can put unnecessary stress on your bones and increase the risk of fractures. Stick to low-impact exercises, such as resistance bands, weights, or stationary cycling.

Avoid twisting and bending: Twisting and bending can put extra pressure on your spine and increase the risk of fractures. Focus on exercises that keep your spine in a neutral position, such as seated rows or chest presses.

Listen to your body: If you experience pain or discomfort during your workout, stop immediately and seek medical attention if necessary. Don't push yourself too hard and always work within your limits.

Consider using equipment: Using equipment such as weightlifting belts, gloves, or wrist wraps can help provide additional support and reduce the risk of injury.

These are just some general safety precautions to consider when doing resistance training for osteoporosis. Always consult with a qualified healthcare professional before starting any new exercise program, and listen to your body to avoid injury

How to progress your resistance training:

Progressing your resistance training is important to ensure that you continue to challenge your muscles and make progress towards your fitness goals. Here are some ways to progress your resistance training:

Increase weight or resistance: As you get stronger, gradually increase the weight or resistance to continue to challenge your muscles. This can be done by adding more weight to dumbbells, using a heavier resistance band, or using heavier weight machines.

Increase reps or sets: If you're not ready to increase the weight or resistance, you can increase the number of reps or sets you do for each exercise. This can help increase your endurance and improve your overall fitness level.

Increase frequency: If you're only doing resistance training once a week, consider adding additional sessions to your weekly routine. This can help increase the overall volume of your workouts and provide more opportunities to challenge your muscles.

Vary your exercises: Incorporating new exercises into your routine can help target different muscle groups and prevent boredom. This can also help prevent plateauing and keep your workouts challenging.

Use different equipment: Trying out new equipment, such as kettlebells or resistance bands, can provide a new challenge and help you progress your resistance training.

Incorporate advanced techniques: Advanced techniques, such as drop sets or super sets, can help challenge your muscles in new ways and provide a greater training stimulus.

5

Chapter 5

Weight-Bearing Exercises:

Definition and benefits of weight-bearing exercises

Osteoporosis is often called the "silent disease" because bone loss can occur without any symptoms or warning signs. Osteoporosis is a significant public health issue, affecting approximately 54 million Americans, with an estimated 10 million Americans over the age of 50 suffering from the disease.

While osteoporosis can affect anyone, it is more common in women, particularly postmenopausal women. This is because estrogen, which is produced by the ovaries, plays an essential role in maintaining bone mass. After menopause, estrogen levels decrease, which can lead to bone loss. Other risk factors for osteoporosis include age, family history, low calcium and vitamin D intake, a sedentary lifestyle, smoking, excessive alcohol consumption, and certain medications.

Weight-bearing exercises, also known as weight-bearing activities, are physical activities that involve bearing one's own body weight through the feet and legs. Examples of weight-bearing exercises include walking, jogging, dancing, stair climbing, and strength training. These exercises are an essential component of any osteoporosis management plan, as they can help improve bone mass, reduce the risk of fractures, and improve overall health and well-being.

We will discuss the definition and benefits of weight-bearing exercises for osteoporosis in more details.

Definition of weight-bearing exercises

Weight-bearing exercises, also known as weight-bearing activities, are physical activities that involve bearing one's own body weight through the feet and legs. These exercises are typically done standing up and can be performed with or without weights. The weight of the body creates resistance against gravity, which stimulates the bones to adapt and become stronger.

There are two types of weight-bearing exercises: high-impact and low-impact. High-impact weight-bearing exercises involve activities that require the feet to leave and touch the ground repeatedly, such as running, jumping, and aerobics. Low-impact weight-bearing exercises involve activities that keep at least one foot on the ground at all times, such as walking, hiking, and dancing. Both types of weight-bearing exercises can help improve bone mass and reduce the risk of fractures, but low-impact exercises are generally safer for individuals with osteoporosis or other conditions that affect bone health, we are are going to discuss about them below.

Benefits of weight-bearing exercises for osteoporosis

Weight-bearing exercises have numerous benefits for individuals with osteoporosis, including:

1. Improving bone mass

Weight-bearing exercises are effective at improving bone mass by stimulating the bone-building cells called osteoblasts. The mechanical stress placed on the bones during weight-bearing exercises causes these cells to become more active, leading to an increase in bone density. Studies have shown that weight-bearing exercises can increase bone mineral density in the hip and spine, which are common fracture sites in individuals with osteoporosis.

2. Reducing the risk of fractures

Weight-bearing exercises can also help reduce the risk of fractures in individuals with osteoporosis. Stronger bones are less likely to fracture, and weight-bearing exercises can help strengthen bones by increasing bone density and improving bone quality. Additionally, weight-bearing exercises can improve balance, coordination, and muscle strength, which can help prevent falls, a leading cause of fractures in older adults.

3. Improving balance and coordination

Weight-bearing exercises can help improve balance and coordination, which are essential for preventing falls. As individuals age, their balance and coordination can deteriorate, increasing their risk of falls and fractures. Weight-bearing exercises can help improve these skills by challenging the body's balance and stability and requiring coordination between different muscle groups.

4. Increasing muscle strength

Weight-bearing exercises can also help increase muscle strength, particularly in the legs and hips. Stronger muscles can help support and protect the bones, reducing the risk of fractures. Additionally, stronger muscles can improve balance and mobility, making daily activities easier and safer to perform.

5. Improving cardiovascular health
Many weight-bearing exercises, such as walking, jogging, and dancing, are also cardiovascular exercises that can improve heart health. Regular cardiovascular exercise can help reduce the risk of heart disease, stroke, and other chronic health conditions, which are more common in individuals with osteoporosis.

6. Improving overall health and well-being
Weight-bearing exercises can also have numerous other health benefits, such as improving mood, reducing stress, and improving sleep quality. Regular exercise can help boost self-esteem and confidence, leading to an overall improved quality of life.

Examples of weight-bearing exercises

They are of two types, high-impact and low-impact:

High impact weight bearing exercises; procedures and time table.

These exercises can help to strengthen bones and improve balance, reducing the risk of falls and fractures. Here are some important high-impact weight-bearing exercises that can be beneficial for people with osteoporosis:

Jumping:

Jumping is an excellent high-impact weight-bearing exercise that can help to build bone density. This can include jumping jacks, jump rope, and plyometric exercises.

Here's a sample daily routine plan for jumping exercises for someone with osteoporosis:

Warm-up:

- Begin with a 5-10 minute warm-up to get your heart rate up and loosen up your muscles.
- This can include light cardio exercises like marching in place, or dynamic stretching exercises.

Jumping jacks:

- Do 3 sets of 10 jumping jacks.
- with a 30-second rest in between sets.
- Make sure to land softly on the balls of your feet, and avoid locking your knees when you land.

Jump rope:

- Do 3 sets of 30 seconds of jump rope, with a 30-second rest in between sets.
- If you don't have a jump rope, you can simulate the motion by jumping in place and swinging your arms as if you were holding a rope.

Plyometric box jumps:

- Find a sturdy box or step and stand in front of it.
- Jump onto the box with both feet, then step back down and repeat for 3 sets of 5 reps.
- If you don't have access to a box, you can do squat jumps instead.

Cool-down:

- Finish your workout with a 5-10 minute cool-down to gradually lower your heart rate and stretch out your muscles.
- This can include static stretching exercises like hamstring stretches, calf stretches, and quadriceps stretches.

Jumping exercises can be challenging for individuals with osteoporosis, as they involve high-impact movements that can put stress on the bones. However, low-impact variations of jumping exercises can still provide benefits without putting excessive strain on the bones. Here is a sample time table for a low-impact jumping routine for someone with osteoporosis:

Monday:

Warm-up: 5 minutes

Low-impact jumping jacks: 2 sets of 10 reps
Rest for 30 seconds
Step-ups on a low bench or stair: 2 sets of 10 reps
Rest for 30 seconds
Toe raises: 2 sets of 10 reps
Cool-down: 5 minutes

Tuesday:

Rest day or gentle stretching exercises

Wednesday:

Warm-up: 5 minutes
Low-impact jumping jacks: 2 sets of 10 reps
Rest for 30 seconds
Knee lifts: 2 sets of 10 reps
Rest for 30 seconds
Lunges with a chair for support: 2 sets of 10 reps
Cool-down: 5 minutes

Thursday:

Rest day or gentle stretching exercises

Friday:

Warm-up: 5 minutes
Low-impact squat jumps: 2 sets of 10 reps
Rest for 30 seconds
Leg swings: 2 sets of 10 reps per leg
Rest for 30 seconds
Calf raises: 2 sets of 10 reps
Cool-down: 5 minutes

Saturday:

Rest day or gentle stretching exercises

Sunday:
  Warm-up: 5 minutes
  Low-impact jumping jacks: 2 sets of 10 reps
  Rest for 30 seconds
  Step-ups with knee lifts on a low bench or stair: 2 sets of 10 reps per leg
  Rest for 30 seconds
  Seated leg extensions with ankle weights: 2 sets of 10 reps per leg
  Cool-down: 5 minutes

It's important to start slowly and gradually increase the intensity and duration of your workouts over time. If you experience any pain or discomfort during the exercises, stop immediately and consult with your healthcare provider

Dancing:

Dancing can be a fun and effective way to build bone density, as it involves high-impact movements that put stress on the bones. Zumba, salsa, and ballroom dancing are all great options.
   Daily routine plan for dancing exercises for someone with osteoporosis:

Warm-up:

- Start with a 5-10 minute warm-up to prepare your body for exercise.
- This can include light cardio exercises such as walking, marching in place, or light dancing movements.

Dance Routine:

- Choose a dance routine that suits your level of fitness and interest.
- You can try salsa, ballroom dancing, Zumba, or any other form of dance that involves high-impact movements such as jumps, hops, and turns.
- Make sure to include weight-bearing exercises such as lunges, squats, and jumps to help improve bone density.

Cool-down:

- End your dance routine with a 5-10 minute cool-down to gradually decrease your heart rate and stretch your muscles.
- This can include gentle stretches, breathing exercises, and relaxation techniques.

Rest and Recovery:

- Give your body time to rest and recover between dance sessions.
- Aim for at least 1-2 days of rest each week to prevent injury and allow your bones and muscles to repair and strengthen.

Consult with a healthcare professional: Before starting any new exercise program, it's important to consult with a healthcare professional to ensure that it is safe for you to do so. They can also provide personalized recommendations and modifications based on your individual needs and abilities.

Remember to listen to your body and modify the exercises as needed to avoid injury. With regular practice and proper guidance, dancing can be a fun and effective way to improve bone density and overall fitness for osteoporosis patients.

Time Table:

Monday:

Warm-up: 5 minutes
  Dancing: 20-30 minutes of ballroom dance
  Strength training: Leg lifts (2 sets of 10 reps)
  Cool-down: 5 minutes

Tuesday:
  Warm-up: 5 minutes
  Dancing: 20-30 minutes of salsa dance
  Strength training: Arm circles (2 sets of 10 reps)
  Cool-down: 5 minutes

Wednesday:
  Rest day or gentle stretching exercises

Thursday:
  Warm-up: 5 minutes
  Dancing: 20-30 minutes of hip hop dance
  Strength training: Squats (2 sets of 10 reps)
  Cool-down: 5 minutes

Friday:
  Warm-up: 5 minutes
  Dancing: 20-30 minutes of ballroom dance
  Strength training: Leg lifts, arm circles, and squats (2 sets of 10 reps each)
  Cool-down: 5 minutes

Saturday:
  Rest day or gentle stretching exercises

Sunday:

Warm-up: 5 minutes

Dancing: 30-40 minutes of a dance style of your choice

Strength training: Leg lifts, arm circles, and squats (3 sets of 10 reps each)

Cool-down: 5 minutes

Remember to listen to your body and make adjustments as needed. If you experience any pain or discomfort during the exercises, stop and consult with a healthcare professional. Also, make sure to choose dance styles and movements that are suitable for your level of fitness and osteoporosis condition.

Running and jogging:

Running and jogging are high-impact weight-bearing exercises that can be effective for building bone density. However, people with osteoporosis should be careful to start slowly and gradually increase the intensity of their workouts.

Daily routine plan for running and jogging exercises:

Warm-up:

- Start with a 5-10 minute warm-up to prepare your body for exercise.
- This can include light cardio exercises such as walking, marching in place, or gentle jumping jacks.

Running and Jogging:

- Choose a safe and flat surface such as a track or treadmill to run or jog on.
- Start with short distances and a slow pace, gradually increasing both

distance and speed over time.
- Avoid running on hard surfaces such as concrete to reduce the risk of stress fractures.

Strength Training:

- Include strength training exercises such as lunges, squats, and calf raises to help improve bone density and reduce the risk of falls.
- This can be done with weights or bodyweight.

Cool-down:

- End your workout with a 5-10 minute cool-down to gradually decrease your heart rate and stretch your muscles.
- This can include gentle stretches and relaxation techniques.

Rest and Recovery:

- Give your body time to rest and recover between workouts.
- Aim for at least 1-2 days of rest each week to prevent injury and allow your bones and muscles to repair and strengthen.

Time Table:

Monday:

Warm-up: 5 minutes

Jogging: 10-15 minutes on a flat surface

Strength training: Squats (2 sets of 10 reps)

Cool-down: 5 minutes

Tuesday:

Warm-up: 5 minutes

Running: 10-15 minutes on a flat surface

Strength training: Wall push-ups (2 sets of 10 reps)

Cool-down: 5 minutes

Wednesday:

Rest day or gentle stretching exercises

Thursday:

Warm-up: 5 minutes

Jogging: 15-20 minutes on a slightly inclined surface

Strength training: Lunges (2 sets of 10 reps)

Cool-down: 5 minutes

Friday:

Warm-up: 5 minutes

Running: 15-20 minutes on a slightly inclined surface

Strength training: Squats, wall push-ups, and lunges (2 sets of 10 reps each)

Cool-down: 5 minutes

Saturday:

Rest day or gentle stretching exercises

Sunday:

Warm-up: 5 minutes
   Jogging: 20-30 minutes on a moderately inclined surface
   Strength training: Squats, wall push-ups, and lunges (3 sets of 10 reps each)
   Cool-down: 5 minutes

Consult with a healthcare professional: you might be wondering why I'm emphasizing on this, but it is very important and necessary to always consult a healthcare professional in any of these activities that will be mentioned below or above please don't be annoyed that I always repeat this same step but make sure that you consult a healthcare professional always.

Hiking:

Hiking is a great way to get weight-bearing exercise while enjoying the outdoors. It can also help to improve balance and coordination.

As mentioned earlier, it's important to consult with a healthcare professional before starting any new exercise routine. However, here is a simple daily routine plan and time table for hiking exercises for someone with osteoporosis:

Daily Routine Plan:

Warm-up:

- Begin with a five to ten-minute warm-up that includes stretching exercises to get your muscles ready for the activity.

Hiking:

- Start with a 10-15 minute hike on a flat surface.
- Increase the duration and intensity gradually as you build up your strength and endurance.

Strength training:

- Perform strength training exercises such as squats, lunges, and wall push-ups to help build bone density and improve balance.
-

Cool-down:

- Finish with a five to ten-minute cool-down that includes stretching exercises to reduce muscle tension and prevent injury.

Time Table:

Monday:
  Warm-up: 5 minutes
  Hiking: 10-15 minutes on a flat surface
  Strength training: Squats (2 sets of 10 reps)
  Cool-down: 5 minutes

Tuesday:
  Warm-up: 5 minutes
  Hiking: 15-20 minutes on a slightly inclined surface
  Strength training: Wall push-ups (2 sets of 10 reps)
  Cool-down: 5 minutes

Wednesday:
Rest day or gentle stretching exercises

Thursday:
Warm-up: 5 minutes
Hiking: 20-30 minutes on a moderately inclined surface
Strength training: Lunges (2 sets of 10 reps)
Cool-down: 5 minutes

Friday:
Warm-up: 5 minutes
Hiking: 30-40 minutes on a challenging surface
Strength training: Squats, wall push-ups, and lunges (2 sets of 10 reps each)
Cool-down: 5 minutes

Saturday:
Rest day or gentle stretching exercises

Sunday:
Warm-up: 5 minutes
Hiking: 40-60 minutes on a challenging surface
Strength training: Squats, wall push-ups, and lunges (3 sets of 10 reps each)
Cool-down: 5 minutes

Stair climbing:

Climbing stairs is a weight-bearing exercise that can help to build bone density in the legs and hips. It can also be a good cardiovascular workout.

Here's a daily routine plan and time table for stair climbing exercises:

Morning:

7:00 AM: Wake up and stretch for 10 minutes.
   7:15 AM: Have a light breakfast.
   8:00 AM: Begin your stair climbing exercises.
   Stair climbing exercise routine:

-
- Start by warming up your muscles with some gentle stretches for 5-10 minutes.
- Begin by climbing one flight of stairs and then walking back down to the bottom.
- Rest for 30 seconds to a minute between each set.
- Repeat this exercise for 3-5 sets, depending on your fitness level and endurance.
- If you feel any discomfort or pain during the exercise, stop immediately and seek medical advice.

Afternoon:

12:00 PM: Have a nutritious lunch.
   1:00 PM: Take a short walk outside, if possible.

Evening:

   5:00 PM: Have a light dinner.
   6:00 PM: Do some light stretching exercises.

7:00 PM: Take a leisurely walk around your neighborhood, if possible. Before Bed:

9:00 PM: Do some gentle stretching to help you relax and unwind before bed.
10:00 PM: Go to bed

Safety precautions for weight-bearing exercises

Here are some safety precautions for weight-bearing exercises for osteoporosis:

Consult with your doctor: It is important to consult with your doctor before starting any new exercise program, especially if you have osteoporosis. Your doctor can advise you on the types of exercises that are safe and appropriate for you.

Start slowly: If you're new to weight-bearing exercises, start slowly and gradually increase the intensity and duration of your exercise routine over time. This will help you avoid injuries and reduce the risk of fractures.

Use proper equipment: Use proper equipment, such as supportive shoes and a sturdy chair, to ensure stability during weight-bearing exercises.

Avoid high-impact exercises: High-impact exercises, such as running or jumping, can increase the risk of fractures for people with osteoporosis. Instead, opt for low-impact exercises, such as walking, stair climbing, or low-impact aerobics.

Incorporate strength training: Strength training exercises, such as weight lifting or resistance band exercises, can help build bone density and reduce the risk of fractures. However, it's important to start with light weights and gradually increase over time.

Maintain good posture: Good posture is important during weight-bearing exercises. Keep your spine straight, your shoulders back, and your core engaged to maintain proper alignment and reduce the risk of injury.

Avoid twisting and bending: Twisting and bending movements can increase the risk of spinal fractures for people with osteoporosis. Avoid exercises that involve excessive twisting or bending, or modify them to reduce the risk of injury

How to progress your weight-bearing exercises

Progressing your weight-bearing exercises is important to continue challenging your body and improving your bone density. Here are some tips on how to progress your weight-bearing exercises:

Increase weight or resistance: Gradually increase the weight or resistance of your exercises over time to continue challenging your muscles and bones. For example, if you're doing bicep curls with 5-pound weights, try increasing to 7-pound weights once you feel comfortable.

Increase repetitions: Increase the number of repetitions of your exercises to build endurance and improve your overall fitness. For example, if you're doing 10 squats, try increasing to 15 squats.

Increase sets: Increase the number of sets of your exercises to continue challenging your body. For example, if you're doing 3 sets of lunges, try increasing to 4 sets.

Increase frequency: Increase the frequency of your weight-bearing exercises to improve your bone density and overall fitness. For example, if you're currently doing weight-bearing exercises 3 times a week, try increasing to 4 or 5 times a week.

Add new exercises: Incorporate new weight-bearing exercises into your routine to continue challenging your body and avoiding boredom. For example, if you're currently doing squats and lunges, try adding in step-ups or calf raises.

Remember to progress your weight-bearing exercises gradually and always listen to your body. If you experience pain or discomfort, stop immediately and consult with your doctor. By progressing your weight-bearing exercises, you can continue improving your bone density and overall health

Low impact weight bearing exercises:

It is important to engage in low-impact exercises to minimize the risk of injury. Here are some examples of low-impact weight-bearing exercises for osteoporosis:

Walking:

Walking is a great low-impact exercise that can help improve bone density. Try to walk for 30 minutes most days of the week.

Dancing:

Dancing is a fun way to get your heart rate up and improve bone density. Look for dance classes that are specifically designed for seniors or those with osteoporosis.

Step aerobics:

Step aerobics can help improve bone density and balance, but it's important to choose a class that is appropriate for your fitness level and avoid high-impact moves.

Yoga:

Yoga can help improve balance, flexibility, and bone density. Look for yoga classes that are designed for seniors or those with osteoporosis.

Resistance training:

Resistance training, using weights or resistance bands, can help improve bone density. It's important to work with a certified personal trainer or physical therapist to develop a safe and effective resistance training program.

CHAPTER 5

Daily routine plan and time table for walking exercises

Here is a sample daily routine plan and time table for walking exercises:

- 6:00 AM - Wake up and do some light stretching exercises to prepare your body for the day.

- 6:30 AM - Start your morning walk. Begin with a 5-10 minute warm-up walk, then increase your pace to a moderate intensity for 30-60 minutes.

- 7:30 AM - Return home and do some cool-down stretches to prevent injury.

- 8:00 AM - Eat a healthy breakfast to refuel your body after your morning walk.

- 9:00 AM - Start your daily activities, whether that be work, school, or other responsibilities.

- 12:00 PM - Take a 10-15 minute walk during your lunch break to get some fresh air and keep your body moving.

- 3:00 PM - Take a quick break from work or other activities to walk around for a few minutes.

- 6:00 PM - Take an evening walk. Begin with a 5-10 minute warm-up walk, then increase your pace to a moderate intensity for 30-60 minutes.

- 7:00 PM - Return home and do some cool-down stretches to prevent injury.

- 8:00 PM – Enjoy a healthy dinner.
-
- 9:00 PM – Wind down for the day with some relaxation exercises like yoga or meditation.
-
- 10:00 PM – Get a good night's sleep to allow your body to rest and recover.

Remember to listen to your body and adjust your walking routine as needed. Also, consult with your doctor or a certified exercise professional if you have any medical conditions that may impact your ability to exercise.

Daily routine plan and time table for dancing exercises

Here is a sample daily routine plan and time table for dancing exercises:

- 6:00 AM – Wake up and do some light stretching exercises to prepare your body for the day.
-
- 6:30 AM – Start your morning with some gentle dance stretches to loosen up your muscles.
-
- 7:00 AM – Eat a healthy breakfast to fuel your body for the day.
-
- 9:00 AM – Start your daily activities, whether that be work, school, or other responsibilities.
-
- 12:00 PM – Take a break from work or other activities to dance to your

favorite music for 10-15 minutes.

-
- 1:00 PM - Eat a healthy lunch to refuel your body.
-
- 3:00 PM - Take a quick dance break for 5-10 minutes to get your blood pumping and boost your energy.
-
- 6:00 PM - Attend a dance class or follow along with a dance workout video for 30-60 minutes.
-
- 7:00 PM - Eat a healthy dinner to replenish your energy.
-
- 8:00 PM - Wind down for the day with some relaxation exercises like yoga or meditation.
-
- 10:00 PM - Get a good night's sleep to allow your body to rest and recover.

Daily routine plan and time table for step acrobatics exercises

Here is a sample daily routine plan and time table for step aerobics exercises:

- 6:00 AM - Wake up and do some light stretching exercises to prepare your body for the day.
-
- 6:30 AM - Start your morning with a 5-10 minute warm-up walk, followed by some gentle step aerobics moves to get your heart rate up and warm up your muscles.

- 7:00 AM - Eat a healthy breakfast to fuel your body for the day.

- 9:00 AM - Start your daily activities, whether that be work, school, or other responsibilities.

12:00 PM - Take a break from work or other activities to do a 10-15 minute step aerobics routine to get your blood pumping and boost your energy.

- 1:00 PM - Eat a healthy lunch to refuel your body.

- 3:00 PM - Take a quick break from work or other activities to do a few minutes of step aerobics to keep your body moving.

- 6:00 PM - Attend a step aerobics class or follow along with a step aerobics workout video for 30-60 minutes.

- 7:00 PM - Eat a healthy dinner to replenish your energy.

- 8:00 PM - Wind down for the day with some relaxation exercises like yoga or meditation.

- 10:00 PM - Get a good night's sleep to allow your body to rest and recover.

CHAPTER 5

Daily routine plan and time table for yoga exercises

Here is a sample daily routine plan and time table for yoga exercises:

- 6:00 AM - Wake up and do some light stretching exercises to prepare your body for the day.
-
- 6:30 AM - Start your morning with some gentle yoga poses to wake up your body and mind.
-
- 7:00 AM - Eat a healthy breakfast to fuel your body for the day.
-
- 9:00 AM - Start your daily activities, whether that be work, school, or other responsibilities.
-
- 12:00 PM - Take a break from work or other activities to do a 10-15 minute yoga routine to relax and re-energize.
-
- 1:00 PM - Eat a healthy lunch to refuel your body.
-
- 3:00 PM - Take a quick break from work or other activities to do a few minutes of yoga to release tension and improve your focus.
-
- 6:00 PM - Attend a yoga class or follow along with a yoga video for 30-60 minutes.
-
- 7:00 PM - Eat a healthy dinner to replenish your energy.
-
- 8:00 PM - Wind down for the day with some relaxation yoga poses and

meditation.
-
- 10:00 PM - Get a good night's sleep to allow your body to rest and recover.

Remember to listen to your body and adjust your yoga routine as needed. It's important to choose a class that is appropriate for your fitness level and avoid poses that may cause discomfort or injury. Also, consult with your doctor or a certified yoga instructor if you have any medical conditions that may impact your ability to practice yoga.

Daily routine plan and time table for resistance training exercises

Here is a sample daily routine plan and time table for resistance training exercises:

- 6:00 AM - Wake up and do some light stretching exercises to prepare your body for the day.
-
- 6:30 AM - Start your morning with a quick 10-15 minute warm-up, such as jogging in place or jumping jacks, to get your blood pumping and warm up your muscles.
-
- 7:00 AM - Eat a healthy breakfast to fuel your body for the day.
-
- 9:00 AM - Start your daily activities, whether that be work, school, or other responsibilities.
-

- 12:00 PM - Take a break from work or other activities to do a 10-15 minute resistance training routine, focusing on different muscle groups each day.

- 1:00 PM - Eat a healthy lunch to refuel your body.

- 3:00 PM - Take a quick break from work or other activities to do a few minutes of resistance training exercises to keep your body moving.

- 6:00 PM - Attend a resistance training class or follow along with a resistance training workout video for 30-60 minutes.

- 7:00 PM - Eat a healthy dinner to replenish your energy.

- 8:00 PM - Wind down for the day with some relaxation exercises like stretching or yoga.

- 10:00 PM - Get a good night's sleep to allow your body to rest and recover.

Chapter 6

Definition and benefits of flexibility and balance exercises:

Flexibility exercises are physical activities that improve the range of motion of your joints and muscles. These exercises typically involve stretching or movement that helps to increase flexibility and reduce muscle stiffness. Flexibility exercises are commonly recommended for people with osteoporosis, as they can help to maintain or improve bone density, reduce the risk of falls, and improve posture.

Types of flexibility exercises

Static stretching:

This involves holding a stretch position for a period of time (usually around 20-30 seconds) without any movement.

CHAPTER 6

Daily routine plan for Static stretching exercises:

Neck Stretch:

- Sit or stand with your arms by your side, and slowly lower your left ear towards your left shoulder.
- Hold for 20-30 seconds, then repeat on the other side.

Shoulder and Upper Back Stretch:

- Sit or stand with your arms by your side, and clasp your hands behind your back.
- Gently pull your hands away from your back and lift your chest. Hold for 20-30 seconds.

Triceps Stretch:

- Extend your right arm overhead and bend your elbow, bringing your hand towards the center of your back.
- Use your left hand to gently push your right elbow back.
- Hold for 20-30 seconds, then repeat on the other side.

Hamstring Stretch:

- Sit on the floor with your legs straight out in front of you.
- Reach forward and try to touch your toes. Hold for 20-30 seconds.

Quadriceps Stretch:

- Stand with your feet hip-width apart, and lift your right heel towards your buttock.
- Hold onto your ankle with your right hand, and gently pull your heel towards your buttock.
- Hold for 20-30 seconds, then repeat on the other side.

Calf Stretch:

- Stand facing a wall, and place your hands on the wall at shoulder height.
- Step your right foot back and press your heel into the floor.
- Hold for 20-30 seconds, then repeat on the other side.

Hip Stretch:

- Lie on your back with your knees bent and your feet flat on the floor.
- Cross your right ankle over your left knee, and gently pull your left knee towards your chest.
- Hold for 20-30 seconds, then repeat on the other side.

Perform each stretch 2-3 times, holding for 20-30 seconds each time. Gradually increase the duration and number of repetitions over time. Remember to breathe deeply and relax into each stretch. If any stretch causes pain, stop immediately and consult with your healthcare provider

Dynamic stretching:

Dynamic stretching exercises involve moving through a range of motion, and can help improve flexibility, balance, and coordination, which are all important for individuals with osteoporosis. Here is a daily routine plan for dynamic stretching exercises for an osteoporosis patient:

Shoulder Circles:

- Stand with your feet hip-width apart and your arms by your side.
- Slowly lift your shoulders towards your ears, then circle them backwards and down.
- Repeat for 10-15 circles, then switch directions.

Arm Swings:

- Stand with your feet hip-width apart and your arms out to the sides.
- Swing your arms forward and then back, crossing them in front of your body and then opening them wide.
- Repeat for 10-15 swings.

Leg Swings:

- Stand with your feet hip-width apart and your hands on your hips.
- Swing your right leg forward and back, keeping it straight.
- Repeat for 10-15 swings, then switch sides.

Knee Lifts:

- Stand with your feet hip-width apart and your arms by your side.

- Lift your right knee towards your chest, then lower it and lift your left knee.
- Repeat for 10-15 lifts on each side.

Ankle Bounces:

- Stand with your feet hip-width apart and your arms by your side.
- Bounce up and down on the balls of your feet, lifting your heels off the ground.
- Repeat for 20-30 bounces.

Side Steps:

- Stand with your feet hip-width apart and take a step to the right with your right foot.
- Bring your left foot to meet your right foot, then step to the left with your left foot.
- Repeat for 10-15 steps in each direction.

Walking Lunges:

- Stand with your feet hip-width apart and your hands on your hips.
- Take a large step forward with your right foot, bending your right knee and keeping your left leg straight.
- Push off with your right foot to bring your left foot forward and repeat on the other side.
- Repeat for 10-15 lunges on each side.

Perform each exercise for 10-15 repetitions, gradually increasing the number over time. Remember to breathe deeply and maintain proper posture throughout each exercise. If any exercise causes pain or discomfort, stop immediately and consult with your healthcare provider

Passive stretching:

This involves using an external force (such as a partner or a stretching aid) to help you stretch.

Passive stretching can be helpful for osteoporosis patients who may have limited mobility and range of motion.

Daily routine plan for passive stretching exercises:

Chest stretch:

- Sit on the edge of a chair with your feet flat on the floor.
- Place your hands behind your head with your elbows pointing out to the sides.
- Gently pull your elbows back and hold the stretch for 20-30 seconds.

Shoulder stretch:

- Stand facing a wall with your arms extended in front of you and your palms flat against the wall.
- Slowly walk your hands up the wall as high as you comfortably can, and hold the stretch for 20-30 seconds.

Hamstring stretch:

- Lie on your back with one leg extended and the other leg bent with your foot flat on the floor.
- Loop a towel or resistance band around the arch of your extended foot and gently pull the leg towards you until you feel a stretch in the back of your thigh.
- Hold for 20-30 seconds, then switch legs.

Quadriceps stretch:

- Stand near a wall or sturdy chair for support.
- Bend one leg at the knee and grab your ankle with your hand, pulling your heel towards your buttocks until you feel a stretch in the front of your thigh.
- Hold for 20-30 seconds, then switch legs.

Calf stretch:

- Stand facing a wall with one foot forward and one foot back.
- Keep your back leg straight and your heel on the ground, and lean forward into the wall until you feel a stretch in your calf. Hold for 20-30 seconds, then switch legs.

Hip flexor stretch:

- Kneel on one knee with the other foot in front of you, making sure your knee is directly above your ankle.
- Slowly lean forward into your front foot until you feel a stretch in your hip flexor.

- Hold for 20-30 seconds, then switch legs.

Perform each stretch for 20-30 seconds, and repeat each stretch 2-3 times. Remember to breathe deeply and hold the stretch without bouncing or overstretching. If any stretch causes pain or discomfort, stop immediately and consult with your healthcare provider.

Active stretching:

Active stretching involves actively contracting and relaxing the muscles being stretched. This type of stretching can help improve flexibility, range of motion, and muscle strength, all of which can be beneficial for osteoporosis patients.

Daily routine plan for active stretching exercises for an osteoporosis patient:

Neck stretch:

- Sit up tall in a chair with your feet flat on the floor.
- Slowly lower your right ear towards your right shoulder, keeping your left shoulder down.
- Hold for a few seconds, then lift your head back to the center.
- Repeat on the other side. Perform 2-3 repetitions on each side.

Shoulder rolls:

- Sit up tall in a chair with your feet flat on the floor.
- Slowly roll your shoulders forwards in a circular motion for 5-10 repetitions, then roll them backwards for another 5-10 repetitions.

Arm circles:

- Stand up straight with your feet hip-width apart.
- Extend your arms straight out to the sides, then make small circles with your arms.
- Gradually increase the size of the circles until you're making big circles.
- Reverse the direction of the circles after 10-15 repetitions.

Hip circles:

- Stand up straight with your feet hip-width apart.
- Place your hands on your hips and make small circles with your hips.
- Gradually increase the size of the circles until you're making big circles.
- Reverse the direction of the circles after 10-15 repetitions.

Knee lifts:

- Stand up straight with your feet hip-width apart.
- Lift your right knee towards your chest, holding onto it with both hands.
- Lower your leg back down to the floor and repeat on the other side.
- Perform 10-15 repetitions on each leg.

Heel raises:

- Stand up straight with your feet hip-width apart.

- Rise up onto your toes, then lower your heels back down to the floor.
- Perform 10-15 repetitions.

Perform each stretch or exercise for 10-15 repetitions, and repeat the entire routine 2-3 times. Remember to breathe deeply and move slowly and smoothly through each stretch or exercise. If any stretch or exercise causes pain or discomfort, stop immediately and consult with your healthcare provider.

Benefits of flexibility exercises for osteoporosis patients:

Improve range of motion: Flexibility exercises can help to improve the range of motion of your joints and muscles, which can help to reduce stiffness and improve mobility. This is particularly important for people with osteoporosis, as it can help to maintain independence and reduce the risk of falls.

Reduce the risk of falls: Falls are a significant risk for people with osteoporosis, as they can lead to fractures and other injuries. Flexibility exercises can help to improve balance and coordination, which can reduce the risk of falls.

Improve posture: Good posture is important for maintaining bone health and reducing the risk of fractures. Flexibility exercises can help to improve posture by reducing muscle tension and improving flexibility in the spine and other areas.

Maintain bone density: Maintaining bone density is important for preventing and managing osteoporosis. Flexibility exercises can help to maintain or improve bone density by promoting the production of new bone tissue.

Definition of balance exercises:

Balance exercises are physical activities that improve your ability to maintain balance and stability. These exercises typically involve standing on one leg, performing movements that challenge your balance, or using balance aids such as stability balls or wobble boards. Balance exercises are particularly beneficial for people with osteoporosis, as they can reduce the risk of falls and improve overall mobility.

Types of balance exercises:

Standing balance exercises:

This involves standing on one leg or performing other movements that challenge your balance.

Here's a daily routine plan for standing balance exercises:

Warm-up:

- Before starting the standing balance exercises, it's important to warm up the body.
- You can do this by walking in place or performing gentle stretches.

Single-leg stance:

- Stand on one leg and hold the position for 30 seconds.
- Repeat with the other leg.
- Start with a stable surface, like a wall or chair, and progress to standing on a less stable surface, like a foam pad.

Tandem stance:

- Stand with one foot in front of the other, heel to toe.
- Hold the position for 30 seconds and then switch the foot in front.
- Use a stable surface for support if needed.

Semi-tandem stance:

- Stand with one foot in front of the other, but with a few inches between the heels.
- Hold the position for 30 seconds and then switch the foot in front.

Clock reach:

- Stand on one foot and reach out with the other foot to touch the numbers of an imaginary clock around you.
- Repeat with the other foot.

Leg swings:

- Stand with feet shoulder-width apart and swing one leg forward and backward, then side-to-side.

- Repeat with the other leg.

- **Heel raises:** Stand with feet shoulder-width apart and raise up onto the balls of your feet.
- Lower down slowly and repeat for 10-15 repetitions.

Toe raises:

- Stand with feet shoulder-width apart and raise up onto your toes.
- Lower down slowly and repeat for 10-15 repetitions.

Cool-down: Finish the routine with a few gentle stretches and breathing exercises.

Dynamic balance exercises:

This involves moving your body through a range of motion while maintaining your balance, such as performing a lunge or squat.

Here's a daily routine plan for dynamic balance exercises for an osteoporosis patient:

Warm-up:

- Before starting the dynamic balance exercises, it's important to warm up the body. You can do this by walking in place or performing gentle stretches.

Single-leg balance with reach:

- Stand on one leg and reach forward with the opposite arm.
- Hold for a few seconds and return to the starting position.
- Repeat with the other leg and arm.

Side-to-side reach:

- Stand with feet shoulder-width apart and reach out to the side with one arm while lifting the opposite leg to the side.
- Return to the starting position and repeat on the other side.

Forward and backward reach:

- Stand with feet shoulder-width apart and reach forward with both arms, then reach backward with both arms.
- Repeat for 10-15 repetitions.

Step-ups:

- Stand in front of a step or sturdy platform and step up with one foot, then bring the other foot up to meet it.
- Step down and repeat with the other foot.
- Use a railing or wall for support if needed.

Lunges:

- Stand with feet shoulder-width apart and step forward with one foot, bending both knees.
- Return to the starting position and repeat with the other foot.
- Use a railing or wall for support if needed.

Side lunges:

- Stand with feet wider than shoulder-width apart and step to the side with one foot, bending the knee while keeping the other leg straight.
- Return to the starting position and repeat on the other side.

Cool-down: Finish the routine with a few gentle stretches and breathing exercises.

Proprioceptive training:

This involves using balance aids such as stability balls or wobble boards to challenge your balance and improve stability.

Here's a daily routine plan for proprioceptive training exercises for an osteoporosis patient:

Warm-up:

- Before starting the proprioceptive training exercises, it's important to warm up the body. You can do this by walking in place or performing gentle stretches.

Single-leg balance with eyes closed:

- Stand on one leg with your eyes closed for 10-15 seconds, then switch to the other leg.
- Use a stable surface for support if needed.

Balance board:

- Stand on a balance board with feet shoulder-width apart and hold the position for 30 seconds.
- Start with a stable board and progress to a more unstable board over time.

Foam pad balance:

- Stand on a foam pad with feet shoulder-width apart and hold the position for 30 seconds.
- Use a stable surface for support if needed.

BOSU ball balance:

- Stand on a BOSU ball with feet shoulder-width apart and hold the position for 30 seconds.
- Use a stable surface for support if needed.

Weight shifting:

- Stand with feet shoulder-width apart and shift your weight from side to side or front to back.
- Start slowly and gradually increase the speed and range of motion.

Wobble board:

- Stand on a wobble board with feet shoulder-width apart and hold the position for 30 seconds.
- Use a stable surface for support if needed.

Cool-down: Finish the routine with a few gentle stretches and breathing exercises.

Benefits of balance exercises for osteoporosis patients:

Reduce the risk of falls: Falls are a significant risk for people with osteoporosis, as they can lead to fractures and other injuries. Balance exercises can help to improve balance and coordination, which can reduce the risk of falls.

Improve overall mobility: Good balance is important for maintaining overall mobility and independence. Balance exercises can help to improve balance and stability, which can make it easier to perform daily activities such as walking, climbing stairs, and getting up from a chair.

Improve bone density: Maintaining bone density is important for preventing and managing osteoporosis. Balance exercises can help to improve bone density by promoting the production of new bone tissue in the areas of the body that are under stress during the exercises.

Improve confidence: Fear of falling can be a significant concern for people with osteoporosis, which can impact their confidence and limit their activities. By improving balance and reducing the risk of falls, balance exercises can help to improve confidence and allow people to participate in activities they might have otherwise avoided.

Benefits of combining flexibility and balance exercises for osteoporosis patients

While both flexibility and balance exercises offer benefits to people with osteoporosis, combining the two can offer even greater benefits. By improving flexibility, people with osteoporosis can improve their range of motion and reduce muscle tension, which can help to improve balance and stability. By improving balance, people with osteoporosis can reduce the risk of falls, which can help to maintain bone health and prevent fractures.

combining flexibility and balance exercises can also help to improve overall fitness levels, reduce stress, and improve overall quality of life. Studies have shown that regular exercise can help to improve mood, reduce anxiety and depression, and increase energy levels.

Flexibility and balance exercises are important components of an exercise program for treating osteoporosis. These exercises can help to improve range of motion, reduce the risk of falls, improve posture, maintain bone density, and improve overall quality of life. By combining flexibility and balance exercises with other forms of exercise such as resistance training and cardiovascular exercise, people with osteoporosis can maintain or improve their physical fitness levels and reduce the risk of fractures and other complications associated with this condition. It is important to work with a healthcare professional or exercise specialist to develop an individualized exercise program that is safe and effective for your individual needs and abilities.

Safety precautions for flexibility and balance training

It is essential to take certain safety precautions to prevent injury during these exercises. Here are some safety tips for flexibility and balance training:

Warm-up: Always begin your flexibility and balance training with a thorough warm-up. This can include light cardio exercises like jogging or jumping jacks, as well as some dynamic stretching.

Progress slowly: When starting a new flexibility or balance exercise, progress slowly to avoid injury. Gradually increase the difficulty level or range of motion as your body adapts to the exercise.

Use proper form: Proper form is crucial for both flexibility and balance exercises. Make sure you understand the correct form before attempting any new exercises. Improper form can lead to muscle strains or falls.

Use support: When first attempting balance exercises, use support such as a wall or chair until you feel more confident. This will help prevent falls.

Wear proper footwear: Make sure you wear shoes that fit well and have good traction when performing balance exercises. This will help prevent slips and falls.

Stay hydrated: Drinking enough water before, during, and after your workout is important to keep your body hydrated and prevent cramping.

Listen to your body: If you feel pain or discomfort during any flexibility or balance exercises, stop immediately. Consult a fitness professional or healthcare provider if necessary

How to progress your flexibility and balance exercises

Progressing your flexibility and balance exercises is important to continue challenging your body and improving your overall fitness.

Tips for progressing your flexibility and balance exercises:

Increase range of motion: When performing flexibility exercises, gradually increase the range of motion. For example, if you are doing a hamstring stretch, try reaching further towards your toes each time.

Hold stretches longer: To improve flexibility, hold your stretches for a longer duration of time. For static stretches, try holding for 30 seconds to one minute.

Incorporate resistance: Adding resistance to your flexibility exercises can help you progress. You can use resistance bands or weights to add extra challenge to your stretches.

Increase duration of balance exercises: To improve your balance, increase the duration of your balance exercises. For example, try holding a one-legged balance for a longer duration each time.

Make balance exercises more challenging: Once you have mastered basic balance exercises, you can make them more challenging. For example, try balancing on an unstable surface such as a foam pad or balance board.

Incorporate dynamic movements: Adding dynamic movements to your balance exercises can help improve your stability and overall body control. For example, try doing squats on a balance board or lunges while holding a weight.

Try new exercises: Incorporating new exercises into your flexibility and balance routine can help keep it fresh and challenging. Try new stretches or balance exercises to keep your body guessing.

Remember to progress slowly and listen to your body. It's important to challenge yourself, but not to the point of pain or discomfort. By gradually increasing the difficulty level of your flexibility and balance exercises, you can continue to improve your overall fitness and achieve your goals of overcoming osteoporosis.

Specific Exercises for Common

Some specific and essential exercises for common areas that people want to improve flexibility and balance:

Hamstrings:

seated forward fold, standing hamstring stretch, lying hamstring stretch, and single-leg hamstring stretch.

Hips:

pigeon pose, hip flexor stretch, butterfly stretch, and fire hydrant exercises.

Shoulders:

shoulder rolls, standing wall stretch, downward dog, and thread-the-needle pose.

Core:

plank, side plank, bridge, and bird dog exercise.

Ankles:

calf raises, ankle rotations, heel-to-toe walk, and balance exercises on an unstable surface.

Knees:

standing quad stretch, seated butterfly stretch, and leg extensions.

Upper back:

cat-cow stretch, seated spinal twist, and cow face pose.

Remember to warm up before stretching and gradually increase the difficulty level of the exercises over time. Additionally, incorporating balance exercises like one-legged stands, lunges, and squats can help improve overall body control and stability. Always listen to your body and stop immediately if you feel any pain or discomfort. It's always a good idea to consult with a fitness professional or healthcare provider before starting any new exercise program.

Chapter 7

Exercises for a better posture and their procedures.

Maintaining good posture is essential for overall health, especially for those with osteoporosis. Here are some exercises to improve posture and daily routines to incorporate them into your daily routine:

Shoulder blade squeeze

Shoulder blade squeeze is a simple exercise that can help improve posture and relieve upper back and shoulder tension. Here are the steps to perform a shoulder blade squeeze exercise:

-
  - Sit or stand with your back straight and your shoulders relaxed.
-
  - Reach both arms straight out in front of you at shoulder height, palms facing down.

- Slowly pull your shoulder blades together and down, squeezing them tightly.

- Hold the squeeze for 5-10 seconds, then release.

- Repeat for 10-15 repetitions.

- As you become more comfortable with the exercise, you can add resistance by holding light weights or using resistance bands.

Remember to breathe slowly and deeply throughout the exercise, and avoid hunching your shoulders or straining your neck. This exercise can be done throughout the day, as needed, to help alleviate tension and improve posture.

Wall angels:

Wall angel is a great exercise for improving upper body posture and mobility, especially in the shoulders and upper back. Here are the steps to perform a wall angel exercise:

- Stand with your back against a wall, with your feet hip-width apart and your knees slightly bent.

- Bring your arms up to a 90-degree angle, with your elbows bent and your palms facing forward. Your upper arms should be parallel to the floor.

- Keeping your arms against the wall, slowly slide your arms up above your head, straightening your elbows as much as you can without lifting your shoulders off the wall.
- Pause briefly at the top, then slowly slide your arms back down to the starting position.
- Repeat for 10-15 repetitions.
- Focus on keeping your back and neck straight, and avoid arching your lower back.

Remember to breathe deeply and maintain good posture throughout the exercise. Wall angel can be done daily, as needed, to improve upper body mobility and posture

Abdominal bracing:

Abdominal bracing is a simple exercise that can help improve core stability and support proper posture. Here are the steps to perform an abdominal bracing exercise:

- Start by lying on your back with your knees bent and your feet flat on the floor.
- Place your hands on your lower abdomen, just below your belly button.

- Take a deep breath in, and as you exhale, gently draw your belly button in towards your spine, as if you are pulling your navel in towards your spine.

- Hold the contraction for 10-15 seconds, keeping your breathing slow and steady.

- Release the contraction and take a few deep breaths before repeating.

- Start with 5-10 repetitions, gradually increasing as you become more comfortable with the exercise

Remember to focus on keeping your lower back flat on the floor and avoid holding your breath or straining your neck. Abdominal bracing can be done daily, as needed, to improve core stability and support proper posture

Hip flexor stretch:

Hip flexor stretch is an effective exercise for stretching the muscles in the front of the hip, which can become tight from prolonged sitting or other activities. Here are the steps to perform a hip flexor stretch:

- Start in a lunge position with your right foot forward and your left foot back.

- Keeping your torso upright, shift your weight forward onto your right foot, bending your knee so that your thigh is parallel to the ground.

- Place your left hand on your left hip for stability, and reach your right arm up overhead.

- Gently tuck your tailbone under and squeeze your glutes to deepen the stretch.

- Hold the stretch for 20-30 seconds, then release and switch sides.

- Repeat 2-3 times on each side.

Remember to breathe deeply and avoid arching your back or leaning forward excessively. Hip flexor stretch can be done daily, as needed, to improve hip flexibility and alleviate tightness in the front of the hip

Walking:

Walking is a low-impact aerobic exercise that can be done by people of all ages and fitness levels. Here are some tips for incorporating walking into your daily routine:

Start with a warm-up: Before you begin your walk, take a few minutes to warm up your muscles with some light stretching or walking at a slower pace.

Set a goal: Whether it's a certain distance, time, or number of steps, setting a goal can help you stay motivated and track your progress.

Choose comfortable shoes: Make sure you wear shoes that fit well and provide adequate support for your feet and ankles.

Maintain good posture: Keep your head up, shoulders relaxed, and arms swinging naturally at your sides.

Increase intensity gradually: If you want to increase the intensity of your walking, do so gradually over time to avoid injury.

Mix it up: Vary your route or terrain to keep your walks interesting, and consider adding some hills or stairs for an added challenge.

Cool down: After your walk, take a few minutes to cool down with some gentle stretching to help prevent muscle soreness and injury.

Remember to listen to your body and adjust your pace or distance as needed. Walking can be done daily, and is a great way to improve cardiovascular health, boost mood, and maintain overall fitness

Standing breaks:

- If you sit for long periods, take breaks every 30 minutes.
- Stand up, stretch, and walk around for a few minutes.
- This will help prevent slouching and improve posture.

By incorporating these exercises and daily routines into your life, you can improve your posture and maintain better overall health, especially if you have osteoporosis. It's important to consult with your healthcare provider before starting any new exercise routine, especially if you have any medical conditions.

8

Chapter 8

Osteoporosis-Related Injuries:

Osteoporosis-related injuries are injuries that occur as a result of weakened bones.
Some of the common types of osteoporosis-related injuries include:

Fractures:

Fractures are the most common type of injury related to osteoporosis. They can occur in different parts of the body, including the spine, hip, wrist, and other bones.

Compression fractures:

Compression fractures are a type of fracture that occurs when the vertebrae in the spine collapse or become compressed. They are a common type of fracture in people with osteoporosis, and they can cause severe pain and mobility problems.

Hip fractures:

Hip fractures are a serious type of injury that can occur in people with osteoporosis. They often require surgery and can lead to long-term disability and reduced quality of life.

Wrist fractures:

Wrist fractures are another common type of injury in people with osteoporosis. They can result from a fall or other trauma, and they can cause pain and difficulty with everyday tasks like writing and opening jars.

Other injuries:

People with osteoporosis are also at increased risk of other types of injuries, including sprains, strains, and dislocations. These injuries can occur in any part of the body and can be very painful and debilitating.

It is important for people with osteoporosis to take steps to prevent injuries, such as maintaining a healthy diet, engaging in regular exercise, and taking medications as prescribed by their doctor. If an injury does occur, prompt treatment and rehabilitation can help to minimize pain and restore function.

Exercises for Compression fractures:

It is important to consult with a healthcare professional before starting any exercise program, as some exercises may not be appropriate for individuals with certain medical conditions.

Here are some exercises that may be beneficial for individuals with compression fractures:
   We have mentioned them earlier.

Walking:

Walking is a low-impact exercise that can help to improve bone density and reduce the risk of falls. Start with short distances and gradually increase the duration and intensity of your walks.

Tai Chi:

Tai Chi is a gentle form of exercise that can help to improve balance, flexibility, and muscle strength. It is also a weight-bearing exercise, which can help to improve bone density.

Water exercises:

Water exercises, such as swimming or water aerobics, are low-impact and can help to improve muscle strength and flexibility. The buoyancy of the water also reduces the pressure on the spine, making it a good exercise option for individuals with compression fractures.

Yoga:

Yoga can help to improve balance, flexibility, and strength, which can reduce the risk of falls and fractures. It is important to avoid poses that put pressure on the spine, such as forward bends, and to use props, such as blocks or straps, as needed to modify poses.

Resistance training:

we have mentioned this earlier, resistance training, such as weightlifting or resistance band exercises, can help to improve bone density and muscle strength. It is important to use light weights and avoid exercises that put pressure on the spine, such as squats or overhead presses.

Exercises for hip fractures:

Here are some exercises that may be beneficial for individuals recovering from a hip fracture:

Range of motion exercises: These exercises can help to improve flexibility and range of motion in the hip joint. Examples include ankle pumps, heel slides, and hip abduction and adduction exercises.

Weight-bearing exercises: Weight-bearing exercises can help to improve bone density and reduce the risk of falls. Examples include walking, hiking, and dancing. It is important to start slowly and gradually increase the intensity of the exercise.

Resistance training: Resistance training can help to improve muscle strength and balance, which can reduce the risk of falls. Examples include squats, lunges, and leg presses. It is important to use light weights and avoid exercises that put too much pressure on the hip joint.

Water exercises: Water exercises, such as swimming or water aerobics, are low-impact and can help to improve muscle strength and flexibility. The buoyancy of the water also reduces the pressure on the hip joint, making it a good exercise option for individuals recovering from a hip fracture.

Balance exercises: Balance exercises can help to improve balance and reduce the risk of falls. Examples include standing on one leg, heel-to-toe walking, and Tai Chi.

Remember to always consult with a healthcare professional before starting any exercise program, especially if you are recovering from a hip fracture. They can help you determine which exercises are safe and effective for you, please do not forget this.

Exercises for vertebral fractures;

Vertebral fractures are a common type of injury in people with osteoporosis, and they can cause severe pain and mobility problems.

Here are some exercises that may be beneficial for individuals with vertebral fractures:
 I have mentioned them earlier.

Walking: Walking is a low-impact exercise that can help to improve bone density and reduce the risk of falls. Start with short distances and gradually increase the duration and intensity of your walks.

Yoga: Yoga can help to improve balance, flexibility, and strength, which can reduce the risk of falls and fractures. It is important to avoid poses that put pressure on the spine, such as forward bends, and to use props, such as blocks or straps, as needed to modify poses.

Resistance training: Resistance training, such as weightlifting or resistance band exercises, can help to improve bone density and muscle strength. It is important to use light weights and avoid exercises that put pressure on the spine, such as squats or overhead presses.

Tai Chi: Tai Chi is a gentle form of exercise that can help to improve balance, flexibility, and muscle strength. It is also a weight-bearing exercise, which can help to improve bone density.

Pilates: Pilates can help to improve core strength and stability, which can reduce the risk of falls and improve posture. It is important to use modifications, such as a foam roller or small ball, to avoid exercises that put pressure on the spine.

Exercises for wrist fractures:

Here are some exercises that may be beneficial for individuals recovering from a wrist fracture:

Range of motion exercises: These exercises can help to improve flexibility and range of motion in the wrist joint. Examples include wrist flexion and extension exercises, wrist rotations, and finger movements.

Grip strengthening exercises: Grip strengthening exercises can help to improve muscle strength in the hand and wrist. Examples include squeezing a stress ball or hand grip, and finger extensions with a rubber band.

Forearm strengthening exercises: Forearm strengthening exercises can help to improve muscle strength and support the wrist. Examples include wrist curls, reverse wrist curls, and forearm rotations with a light weight.

Modified push-ups: Modified push-ups can help to strengthen the muscles in the chest, shoulders, and arms, which can help to support the wrist during daily activities. Examples include wall push-ups or push-ups on the knees.

Cardiovascular exercises: Cardiovascular exercises, such as walking, cycling, or swimming, can help to improve overall fitness and reduce the risk of future injuries. It is important to start slowly and gradually increase the intensity of the exercise.

Exercises for other common osteoporosis-related injuries:

In addition to the specific exercises mentioned above for compression fractures, hip fractures, vertebral fractures, and wrist fractures, there are some exercises that may be beneficial for other common osteoporosis-related injuries, such as:

Ankle fractures:
Range of motion exercises, such as ankle circles and toe raises, can help to improve flexibility and range of motion in the ankle joint. Weight-bearing

exercises, such as walking or using an elliptical machine, can help to improve bone density and reduce the risk of future fractures. Strengthening exercises for the calf muscles, such as heel raises, can also be beneficial.

Shoulder fractures:

Range of motion exercises, such as arm circles and shoulder shrugs, can help to improve flexibility and range of motion in the shoulder joint. Strengthening exercises for the rotator cuff muscles, such as external rotations with a resistance band, can help to improve stability and reduce the risk of future injuries. Modified push-ups and chest presses can also be beneficial for strengthening the muscles in the chest, shoulders, and arms.

Rib fractures:

Gentle breathing exercises, such as diaphragmatic breathing, can help to improve lung function and reduce pain during breathing. It is also important to avoid activities that put pressure on the ribs, such as heavy lifting or twisting, until the fractures have healed.

9

Chapter 9

Overcoming Barriers to Exercise:

Common barriers to exercise and how to overcome them.

Exercise can help improve bone density, balance, and overall strength, which can reduce the risk of falls and fractures. However, there are some common barriers that may prevent individuals with osteoporosis from engaging in regular exercise. Here are some of these barriers and ways to overcome them:

Fear of falls and fractures: Individuals with osteoporosis may fear that exercising can increase their risk of falls and fractures. To overcome this barrier, it is essential to choose exercises that are safe and appropriate for their condition. Low-impact exercises such as walking, swimming, and cycling can be beneficial for improving bone density and reducing the risk of falls.

Lack of knowledge and guidance: Some individuals with osteoporosis may lack knowledge of safe and effective exercise techniques for their condition.

They may also lack guidance from a healthcare professional or qualified exercise specialist. To overcome this barrier, it is important to seek guidance from a healthcare professional or qualified exercise specialist who can develop an appropriate exercise program tailored to their individual needs.

Pain and discomfort: Individuals with osteoporosis may experience pain and discomfort when exercising, which can discourage them from continuing with their exercise routine. To overcome this barrier, it is important to start with low-impact exercises that are less likely to cause pain and discomfort. Gradually increasing the intensity and duration of exercise can help individuals build up their strength and tolerance.

Time constraints: Some individuals with osteoporosis may feel that they do not have enough time to exercise regularly. To overcome this barrier, it is important to set realistic goals and prioritize exercise as a part of their daily routine. Shorter sessions of exercise, such as 10-15 minutes, can be effective for improving bone density and reducing the risk of falls.

Lack of motivation: Lack of motivation can be a common barrier for individuals with osteoporosis, particularly if they do not see immediate results. To overcome this barrier, it is important to find an exercise routine that is enjoyable and sustainable. Exercise programs that include social support, such as group fitness classes or exercise buddies, can help to maintain motivation and adherence.

Individuals with osteoporosis may face several barriers to engaging in regular exercise. However, with appropriate guidance, education, and support, it is possible to overcome these barriers and incorporate safe and effective exercise into their daily routine.

How to stay motivated to exercise:

Staying motivated to exercise can be a challenge, especially when life gets busy or when progress seems slow. There are several strategies that can help you stay motivated and committed to your exercise routine:

Set realistic goals: Setting achievable goals can help you stay motivated and give you a sense of accomplishment when you reach them. Make sure your goals are specific, measurable, and time-bound, and break them down into smaller milestones to track your progress along the way.

Find activities you enjoy: Choose activities that you enjoy and look forward to, whether it's dancing, hiking, yoga, or swimming. This can make exercise feel less like a chore and more like a fun activity.

Mix it up: Doing the same exercise routine day after day can get boring and lead to burnout. Try different types of exercise or switch up your routine to keep it interesting and challenging.

Exercise with a friend or group: Exercising with a friend or joining a fitness group can help you stay accountable and motivated. It can also make exercise more enjoyable and social.

Reward yourself: Set up a reward system for yourself when you reach a certain milestone or achieve a specific goal. This can help motivate you to keep going and give you something to look forward to.

Focus on the benefits: Remind yourself of the benefits of exercise, such as improved physical health, increased energy, reduced stress, and improved mood. This can help you stay motivated and committed to your exercise routine.

Make exercise a habit: Incorporate exercise into your daily routine and make it a habit. Start small, with short workouts or brief walks, and gradually increase the duration and intensity over time.

Remember, staying motivated to exercise is a journey, not a destination. It's normal to experience setbacks and challenges along the way. By using these strategies and staying committed to your goals, you can stay motivated and enjoy the benefits of regular exercise which you will in turn overcome osteoporosis.

Strategies for finding time to exercise:

Finding time to exercise can be challenging, especially if you have a busy schedule or many responsibilities. However, there are several strategies that can help you prioritize exercise and make it a part of your routine:

Schedule exercise into your day: Treat exercise like any other appointment or commitment and schedule it into your day. Choose a time that works best for you, whether it's first thing in the morning, during your lunch break, or in the evening.

Multitask: Look for ways to combine exercise with other activities, such as walking or biking to work, doing squats or lunges while watching TV, or taking a fitness class with a friend.

Break it up: You don't have to do all your exercise at once. Try breaking it up into shorter sessions throughout the day, such as taking a 10-minute walk during your lunch break or doing a 15-minute workout before work.

Prioritize: Consider what activities you can cut back on or eliminate to make time for exercise. For example, could you spend less time watching TV or scrolling through social media to make time for a workout?

Get up earlier: Consider waking up earlier to make time for exercise before your day gets busy. Even a 20-30 minute workout can be effective for improving your fitness and energy levels.

Make it a family activity: Involve your family or friends in your exercise routine by taking a walk together, playing a game of basketball, or doing a workout class together.

Use your commute: If you have a long commute, consider using it as an opportunity to exercise. Take the stairs instead of the elevator or walk part of the way to work.

Remember, finding time to exercise is about making it a priority and finding ways to incorporate it into your daily routine. By using these strategies and staying committed to your goals, you can make exercise a regular part of your life.

Strategies for finding time to exercise:

Finding time to exercise can be challenging, especially if you have a busy schedule or many responsibilities. There are several strategies that can help you prioritize exercise and make it a part of your routine:

Schedule exercise into your day: Treat exercise like any other appointment or commitment and schedule it into your day. Choose a time that works best for you, whether it's first thing in the morning, during your lunch break, or in the evening.

Multitask: Look for ways to combine exercise with other activities, such as walking or biking to work, doing squats or lunges while watching TV, or taking a fitness class with a friend.

Break it up: You don't have to do all your exercise at once. Try breaking it up into shorter sessions throughout the day, such as taking a 10-minute walk during your lunch break or doing a 15-minute workout before work.

Prioritize: Consider what activities you can cut back on or eliminate to make time for exercise. For example, could you spend less time watching TV or scrolling through social media to make time for a workout?

Get up earlier: Consider waking up earlier to make time for exercise before your day gets busy. Even a 20-30 minute workout can be effective for improving your fitness and energy levels.

Make it a family activity: Involve your family or friends in your exercise routine by taking a walk together, playing a game of basketball, or doing a workout class together.

Use your commute: If you have a long commute, consider using it as an opportunity to exercise. Take the stairs instead of the elevator or walk part of the way to work.

CHAPTER 9

How to adjust your exercise routine for physical limitations:

Exercise is an important part of managing osteoporosis, but it's important to adjust your exercise routine to accommodate any physical limitations.

Here are some tips for adjusting your exercise routine for physical limitations due to osteoporosis:

Consult with your doctor or physical therapist: Before starting any exercise program, it's important to consult with your doctor or physical therapist to determine which exercises are safe and appropriate for you.

Focus on weight-bearing exercises: Weight-bearing exercises can help improve bone density and strength. Examples of weight-bearing exercises include walking, hiking, dancing, and stair climbing.

Modify high-impact exercises: High-impact exercises such as running or jumping can increase the risk of fractures. Instead, consider modifying these exercises to reduce the impact, such as by using a low-impact elliptical machine or performing jumping jacks with a lower intensity.

Incorporate strength training: Strength training can help improve bone density and strength, but it's important to start slowly and gradually increase the weight and intensity of the exercises. Consider using resistance bands, free weights, or weight machines.

Practice balance exercises: Osteoporosis can increase the risk of falls, so it's important to incorporate balance exercises to improve stability and reduce the risk of falls. Examples of balance exercises include yoga, tai chi, and standing on one leg.

Use caution with twisting and bending: Twisting and bending can increase the risk of fractures in people with osteoporosis. When performing exercises that involve twisting or bending, be sure to use caution and avoid overexertion.

Stay hydrated: Adequate hydration is important for maintaining healthy bones, so be sure to drink plenty of water before, during, and after exercise.

Remember to always listen to your body and stop any exercise that causes pain or discomfort. With the right adjustments

Consider low-impact exercises: Low-impact exercises such as swimming, cycling, and using an elliptical machine can be easier on the joints and reduce the risk of injury.

Stretching: Stretching can help improve flexibility, range of motion, and reduce the risk of injury. It's important to stretch before and after exercise, and to perform stretches that target the major muscle groups.

Avoid excessive spinal flexion: People with osteoporosis are at increased risk of spinal fractures, so it's important to avoid excessive spinal flexion or bending forward. Avoid exercises such as sit-ups, crunches, and toe touches, which can place undue stress on the spine.

Use appropriate footwear: Proper footwear is important for reducing the risk of falls and injuries. Choose shoes that provide good support and have a non-slip sole.

Be consistent: Regular exercise is important for maintaining bone health and improving overall fitness. Aim to exercise for at least 30 minutes a day, most days of the week, and gradually increase the duration and intensity of your workouts.

10

Chapter 10

Living Strong with Osteoporosis:

The importance of ongoing exercise for osteoporosis management:

Exercise is an important part of managing osteoporosis, but it's important to adjust your exercise routine to accommodate any physical limitations.

Below are some tips for adjusting your exercise routine for physical limitations due to osteoporosis:

Consult with your doctor or physical therapist: Before starting any exercise program, it's important to consult with your doctor or physical therapist to determine which exercises are safe and appropriate for you.

Focus on weight-bearing exercises: Weight-bearing exercises can help improve bone density and strength. Examples of weight-bearing exercises include walking, hiking, dancing, and stair climbing.

Modify high-impact exercises: High-impact exercises such as running or jumping can increase the risk of fractures. Instead, consider modifying these exercises to reduce the impact, such as by using a low-impact elliptical machine or performing jumping jacks with a lower intensity.

Incorporate strength training: Strength training can help improve bone density and strength, but it's important to start slowly and gradually increase the weight and intensity of the exercises. Consider using resistance bands, free weights, or weight machines.

Practice balance exercises: Osteoporosis can increase the risk of falls, so it's important to incorporate balance exercises to improve stability and reduce the risk of falls. Examples of balance exercises include yoga, tai chi, and standing on one leg.

Use caution with twisting and bending: Twisting and bending can increase the risk of fractures in people with osteoporosis. When performing exercises that involve twisting or bending, be sure to use caution and avoid overexertion.

Stay hydrated: Adequate hydration is important for maintaining healthy bones, so be sure to drink plenty of water before, during, and after exercise.

Consider low-impact exercises: Low-impact exercises such as swimming, cycling, and using an elliptical machine can be easier on the joints and reduce the risk of injury.

Stretching: Stretching can help improve flexibility, range of motion, and reduce the risk of injury. It's important to stretch before and after exercise, and to perform stretches that target the major muscle groups.

Avoid excessive spinal flexion: People with osteoporosis are at increased risk of spinal fractures, so it's important to avoid excessive spinal flexion or bending forward. Avoid exercises such as sit-ups, crunches, and toe touches, which can place undue stress on the spine.

Use appropriate footwear: Proper footwear is important for reducing the risk of falls and injuries. Choose shoes that provide good support and have a non-slip sole.

Be consistent: Regular exercise is important for maintaining bone health and improving overall fitness. Aim to exercise for at least 30 minutes a day, most days of the week, and gradually increase the duration and intensity of your workouts.

The importance of ongoing exercise for osteoporosis management:

Ongoing exercise is an essential component of managing osteoporosis. Regular physical activity helps to maintain and improve bone density, strength, and balance, which can reduce the risk of falls and fractures. Exercise also has many other health benefits, including improving cardiovascular health, reducing the risk of chronic diseases such as diabetes and obesity, and promoting overall physical and mental well-being.

Specific ways in which ongoing exercise can help manage osteoporosis:

Builds bone density: Weight-bearing and resistance exercises help to build bone density and strength, which is particularly important for people with osteoporosis, who have a higher risk of fractures.

Improves balance and reduces falls: Exercise that incorporates balance and coordination training, such as yoga, tai chi, or Pilates, can improve balance and reduce the risk of falls. This is particularly important for older adults with osteoporosis, who are at increased risk of falls and fractures.

Reduces pain: Exercise can help to reduce pain associated with osteoporosis and improve overall quality of life.

Helps maintain a healthy weight: Regular physical activity can help to maintain a healthy weight, which is important for reducing the risk of osteoporosis and other chronic diseases.

Promotes overall physical and mental well-being: Exercise has been shown to improve mood, reduce stress, and promote overall physical and mental well-being.

It's important to note that ongoing exercise does not have to be intense or time-consuming to be effective. Even light to moderate exercise, sell-beinglking or gardening, can provide health benefits. The key is to find an exercise routine that is enjoyable, safe, and sustainable for the individual.

Improves flexibility and range of motion: Regular exercise, particularly stretching and flexibility exercises, can improve joint flexibility and range of motion. This can help to reduce stiffness and pain associated with osteoporosis.

Enhances muscle strength: Resistance training exercises, such as weight lifting or using resistance bands, can help to improve muscle strength. This is important for maintaining balance, reducing the risk of falls, and improving overall physical function.

Supports joint health: Regular exercise can help to support joint health by improving circulation, promoting the delivery of nutrients and oxygen to the joints, and reducing inflammation.

Improves sleep quality: Exercise has been shown to improve sleep quality and reduce the risk of insomnia. This is particularly important for people with osteoporosis, who may experience sleep disturbances due to pain or other symptoms.

Boosts self-esteem and confidence: Regular exercise can help to boost self-esteem and confidence, particularly when progress is made in achieving fitness goals. This can have a positive impact on overall well-being and quality of life.

Ongoing exercise is a critical component of managing osteoporosis and promoting overall health and well-being. It has numerous benefits, including building bone density and strength, improving balance and reducing falls, reducing pain, enhancing flexibility and range of motion, and boosting self-esteem and confidence.

How to track your progress and set new goals

Tracking your progress and setting new goals is an important part of maintaining a successful exercise program for osteoporosis management.
Steps to help you track your progress and set new goals:

Keep a workout journal: Keep a journal to record your workouts, including the exercises you did, the sets and reps, and the weight or resistance used. This will help you to monitor your progress over time and see where you have made improvements.

Measure your fitness level: Measure your fitness level periodically, such as every 6 months or annually, to see how your overall fitness has improved. This can include tests such as a timed walk or run, balance tests, or strength assessments.

Use a pedometer or fitness tracker: Use a pedometer or fitness tracker to monitor your daily steps, activity levels, and calories burned. This can help you to set realistic goals and track your progress.

Set new goals: Once you have achieved your initial exercise goals, set new ones to continue improving. For example, you may want to increase the weight or resistance used in your resistance training exercises, improve your balance, or complete a longer-distance walk or run.

Make your goals specific, measurable, achievable, relevant, and time-bound (SMART): SMART goals are specific, measurable, achievable, relevant, and time-bound. This means that your goals should be specific and focused, measurable so you can track progress, achievable with a realistic timeframe, relevant to your needs and interests, and time-bound with a set deadline.

Celebrate your successes: Celebrate your successes along the way to keep yourself motivated and on track. This can include treating yourself to something you enjoy, such as a favorite healthy meal or a new workout outfit.

Please do not forget to always work with your healthcare provider or a certified exercise professional to develop a safe and effective exercise program that meets your individual needs and limitations. By tracking your progress and setting new goals, you can continue to improve your bone health, reduce the risk of falls and fractures, and improve your overall health and well-being.

Success stories of individuals with osteoporosis who have improved their bone health through exercise:

Osteoporosis affects an estimated 200 million women worldwide. However, there are success stories of individuals with osteoporosis who have improved their bone health through exercise. Below, we'll explore some of these success stories and how exercise has helped them manage their condition.

Let's take a look at some success stories of individuals with osteoporosis who have improved their bone health through exercises.

Joanne, 65 years old

Joanne was diagnosed with osteoporosis in her early sixties. Her doctor recommended that she begin taking medication to slow the progression of her condition. However, Joanne was wary of the potential sideyeffects of medication and was keen to explore alternative options. She began researching the benefits of exercise for people with osteoporosis and decided to start a regular exercise routine.

Joanne began by walking for 30 minutes a day and gradually increased the intensity of her workouts by adding resistance training using weights. Over time, she noticed an improvement in her bone density and overall fitness. She also noticed that her balance and coordination had improved, reducing her risk of falls.

Today, Joanne continues to exercise regularly, incorporating a mix of cardio and strength training exercises into her routine. She's delighted with the progress she's made and feels confident that her bone health has improved significantly.

Susan, 70 years old

Susan was diagnosed with osteoporosis in her late sixties. She was initially hesitant to begin an exercise routine as she was concerned about the potential risk of falls. However, her doctor recommended that she start a gentle exercise routine and provided her with guidance on how to exercise safely.

Susan began by incorporating low-impact exercises into her routine, such as swimming, walking, and yoga. She also started lifting weights, but with a lighter weight than what she used to lift. Over time, she noticed an improvement in her strength, flexibility, and balance.

Susan now exercises for 45 minutes a day, five days a week, and has noticed a significant improvement in her bone density. She feels more confident in her ability to move safely and is delighted with the progress she's made.

John, 75 years old

John was diagnosed with osteoporosis in his early seventies. He was initially prescribed medication, but he experienced some side effects, and his doctor recommended that he explore other options. John had always been active, but he hadn't been exercising regularly in recent years.

John began by incorporating low-impact exercises such as cycling, walking, and swimming into his routine. He also began lifting weights, focusing on his lower body, which is where he was at the highest risk of fractures. Over time, John noticed that his bone density had improved, and he felt more confident in his ability to move safely.

John now exercises for an hour a day, six days a week, and incorporates a mix of cardio and strength training exercises into his routine. He's delighted with the progress he's made and feels that exercise has played a significant role in managing his osteoporosis.

Maria, 60 years old

Maria was diagnosed with osteoporosis in her mid-fifties. She had always been active, but she noticed that her bone density was decreasing despite her active lifestyle. She decided to seek the advice of a physical therapist who specialized in working with people with osteoporosis.

The physical therapist recommended a combination of weight-bearing exercises, resistance training, and balance exercises to help improve Maria's bone density and reduce her risk of falls. Maria also worked on her posture, as she had a slight curvature of the spine.

Maria began by incorporating walking, hiking, and weightlifting into her routine. She also practiced balance exercises such as standing on one leg and using a stability ball. Over time, Maria noticed an improvement in her bone density, and her posture had improved significantly.

Maria now exercises for 45 minutes a day, five days a week, and continues to work with her physical therapist to monitor her progress. She feels more confident in her ability to move safely and is delighted with the progress she's made.

Bill, 80 years old

Bill was diagnosed with osteoporosis in his late seventies. He had always been active, but he had stopped exercising regularly due to his age and some health issues. However, he was determined to improve his bone health and decided to start a regular exercise routine.

Bill began by incorporating low-impact exercises such as walking and cycling into his routine. He also started lifting weights, focusing on his upper body, as he had some mobility issues in his lower body. Over time, Bill noticed an improvement in his strength and overall fitness.

Bill now exercises for 30 minutes a day, five days a week, and has noticed a significant improvement in his bone density. He feels more confident in his ability to move safely and is delighted with the progress he's made.

These success stories show that exercise can be an effective way to improve bone health in people with osteoporosis. Regular exercise, including weight-bearing exercises, resistance training, and balance exercises, can help improve bone density, reduce the risk of falls, and improve overall fitness. It's essential to consult with a healthcare professional before starting an exercise routine, especially if you have a medical condition. A physical therapist can also provide guidance on safe and effective exercises for people with osteoporosis.

While osteoporosis can be a debilitating condition, it doesn't have to be a barrier to an active and healthy lifestyle. With the right exercise routine, people with osteoporosis can significantly improve their bone health and reduce the risk of fractures. These success stories are an inspiration to anyone looking to improve their bone health through exercise.

Resources for continuing your osteoporosis exercise routine:

Prominent resources to help you continue your osteoporosis exercise routine:

National Osteoporosis Foundation: The National Osteoporosis Foundation has resources for exercise and physical activity to help prevent and manage osteoporosis. Their website includes videos and guides on exercises for bone health, balance and falls prevention, and low-impact activities.

American Council on Exercise: The American Council on Exercise provides information on exercise for people with osteoporosis. They offer a certified speciality program for fitness professionals called "Bone Health and Osteoporosis" that can help you find a qualified trainer in your area.

The Osteoporosis Society: The Osteoporosis Society is a UK-based charity that provides information on osteoporosis, including resources on exercise and physical activity. They have guides on exercises that are safe and effective for people with osteoporosis, as well as information on the benefits of exercise for bone health.

International Osteoporosis Foundation: The International Osteoporosis Foundation provides information on exercise and physical activity for people with osteoporosis. They have resources on exercises for bone health, as well as information on the importance of a healthy diet and lifestyle.

YouTube: YouTube is a great resource for finding exercise videos specifically designed for people with osteoporosis. Some popular channels that offer osteoporosis-friendly exercises include "Sit and Be Fit," "Fitness Blender," and "Yoga with Adriene."

Physical Therapy: A physical therapist can help you create an exercise plan that is tailored to your specific needs and goals. They can also teach you proper form and technique to help prevent injury and ensure that you are getting the most benefit from your exercises. You can ask your doctor for a referral to a physical therapist who specializes in osteoporosis.

Local Community Centers: Many local community centers offer exercise classes specifically designed for people with osteoporosis. These classes may include activities such as yoga, tai chi, or low-impact aerobics. Check with your local community center or senior center to see what classes are available.

Walking: Walking is a low-impact exercise that can help improve bone density and overall health. Consider taking daily walks around your neighborhood or local park. Start with shorter walks and gradually increase your distance and pace over time.

Strength Training: Strength training can help improve bone density and muscle strength, which can reduce the risk of falls and fractures. Consider incorporating strength training exercises, such as weight lifting or resistance band exercises, into your routine. It's important to work with a qualified trainer or physical therapist to ensure that you are using proper form and technique.

Stay Motivated: It can be challenging to stay motivated to exercise, especially if you are dealing with pain or other health issues. Consider enlisting the support of friends or family members to exercise with you, or join a support group for people with osteoporosis. You can also track your progress and set achievable goals to help stay motivated.

Remember, consistency is key when it comes to exercise and bone health. Incorporating regular exercise into your routine can help improve bone density and reduce the risk of fractures. Be patient and stay committed to your exercise plan, and you'll soon see the benefits of your hard work!!!!!!!!

11

Chapter 11

Lifestyle Changes to Support Bone Health:

Nutrition for bone health:

Nutrition plays a crucial role in maintaining and supporting bone health. Here are some key nutrients that are important for bone health:

Calcium:

Calcium is the most important nutrient for bone health, as it provides the building blocks for bone tissue. Good sources of calcium include dairy products, leafy green vegetables, fortified foods, and supplements.

Vitamin D:

Vitamin D helps the body absorb calcium and supports bone growth and development. It can be found in fatty fish, egg yolks, and fortified foods. The body also produces vitamin D when exposed to sunlight.

Magnesium:

Magnesium is essential for the absorption and metabolism of calcium. It can be found in nuts, whole grains, and green leafy vegetables.

Vitamin K:

Vitamin K plays a role in bone formation and may help improve bone density. Good sources of vitamin K include leafy green vegetables, broccoli, and Brussels sprouts.

Protein:

Protein is important for bone health, as it provides the structural framework for bones. Good sources of protein include lean meats, fish, eggs, and beans.

Phosphorus:

Phosphorus is a mineral that works with calcium to support bone health. It can be found in dairy products, meat, fish, and whole grains.

It is important to consume a balanced diet that includes these key nutrients to support bone health. If you are unable to meet your nutrient needs through diet alone, supplements may be recommended by your healthcare provider.

Excessive intake of certain nutrients, such as vitamin A and vitamin E, may have negative effects on bone health, so it is important to speak with your healthcare provider before taking any supplements

Other lifestyle changes that can support bone health

There are other lifestyle changes and habits that can support bone health. Here are some examples:

Engage in weight-bearing exercises: Weight-bearing exercises such as walking, jogging, dancing, and weightlifting help to build and maintain bone density. Aim for at least 30 minutes of weight-bearing exercise most days of the week.

Practice balance exercises: Balance exercises such as yoga, tai chi, and Pilates can help improve balance and prevent falls, which can lead to fractures.

Quit smoking: Smoking is associated with a higher risk of osteoporosis and bone fractures. Quitting smoking can help improve bone health.

Limit alcohol consumption: Drinking too much alcohol can reduce bone density and increase the risk of fractures. Limit your alcohol intake to no more than one drink per day for women and two drinks per day for men.

Manage stress: Chronic stress can increase the production of cortisol, a hormone that can weaken bones over time. Find ways to manage stress, such as meditation, yoga, or deep breathing exercises.

Get enough sleep: Sleep is important for bone health, as it is during sleep that bones undergo repair and regeneration. Aim for 7-8 hours of sleep per night

The importance of calcium and vitamin D:

Calcium and vitamin D are two of the most important nutrients for bone health. Calcium is a mineral that is essential for building and maintaining strong bones, while vitamin D helps the body absorb calcium and supports bone growth and development.

Calcium:

Calcium is the primary component of bone tissue, making up about 99% of the body's calcium. When the body doesn't get enough calcium through the diet, it may start to take calcium from the bones, which can lead to weaker bones over time. Therefore, it is important to consume enough calcium to maintain bone health. Good sources of calcium include dairy products, leafy green vegetables, fortified foods, and supplements.

Vitamin D:

Vitamin D is essential for calcium absorption in the gut and plays a crucial role in bone development and maintenance. Without enough vitamin D, the body cannot effectively absorb calcium from the diet, leading to weaker bones over time. Vitamin D can be found in fatty fish, egg yolks, and fortified foods. The body also produces vitamin D when exposed to sunlight.

It is recommended that adults get 1,000 to 1,200 milligrams of calcium per day and 600 to 800 International Units (IU) of vitamin D per day. However, individual needs may vary based on factors such as age, sex, and overall health status. It is important to talk to your healthcare provider about your specific nutrient needs and any supplements you may need to support bone health

Limiting risk factors for osteoporosis:

Here are some ways to limit risk factors for osteoporosis and by quitting some harmful addictions.

Please you can do it there is no addiction that is impossible to conquer!!!!!!!!

Quit smoking: Smoking is associated with a higher risk of osteoporosis and fractures. Quitting smoking can help improve bone health.

Limit alcohol consumption: Drinking too much alcohol can reduce bone density and increase the risk of fractures. Limit your alcohol intake to no more than one drink per day for women and two drinks per day for men.

Get enough calcium and vitamin D: As mentioned earlier, calcium and vitamin D are essential nutrients for bone health. Consuming enough calcium and vitamin D through the diet or supplements can help maintain bone health and reduce the risk of osteoporosis.

Engage in weight-bearing and strength-training exercises: Weight-bearing exercises, such as walking, jogging, and dancing, and strength-training exercises, such as lifting weights, can help improve bone density and reduce the risk of fractures.

Avoid falls: Falls can increase the risk of fractures, especially in older adults. To reduce the risk of falls, make sure your home is free of hazards, such as loose rugs or clutter, and use assistive devices, such as handrails or grab bars.

Manage medications: Some medications, such as corticosteroids and certain anticonvulsants, can increase the risk of osteoporosis. If you are taking medications that may affect bone health, talk to your healthcare provider about ways to manage this risk.

By taking steps to limit these risk factors, you can help maintain bone health and reduce the risk of osteoporosis and fractures. It is important to talk to your healthcare provider about your individual risk factors and any steps you can take to maintain bone health

12

Conclusion

In conclusion, "Stronger Bones, Stronger You: A Complete Guide to Exercise for Osteoporosis" provides valuable information and practical guidance for anyone looking to build and maintain healthy bones at any age. By understanding osteoporosis and the benefits of exercise, readers can take proactive steps to manage their bone health and reduce the risk of fractures and other complications.

With clear explanations of the types of exercises recommended for osteoporosis, safety tips, and specific exercises for common injuries, this book empowers readers to develop a safe and effective exercise plan that works for their individual needs and goals.

The importance of lifestyle changes, such as nutrition and limiting risk factors, is also highlighted, emphasizing the need for a holistic approach to bone health. Additionally, the book provides strategies for overcoming barriers to exercise and staying motivated to continue a routine that can improve bone health.

Ultimately, "Stronger Bones, Stronger You" is a comprehensive guide that can help anyone with osteoporosis take control of their bone health and live a stronger, more active life. By following the advice and tips in this book and the success stories found in this book which will serve as a motivation, readers can achieve improved bone density, better posture, increased flexibility and balance, and ultimately a greater sense of wellbeing.

It is more than just a book, "Stronger Bones, Stronger You" is a resource for lifelong bone health. By incorporating the exercises and lifestyle changes outlined in this guide into your daily routine, you can not only prevent further bone loss but also improve your overall quality of life.

Remember, it is never too late to start taking care of your bones. Whether you have recently been diagnosed with osteoporosis or simply want to maintain healthy bones as you age, this book is an excellent starting point. With commitment and dedication, you can make significant strides towards building stronger bones and living a happier, healthier life.

So why wait? Start reading "Stronger Bones, Stronger You" today and take the first step towards a stronger, healthier you.